CRAM SESSION IN

Functional
Neuroanatomy

A Handbook for Students & Clinicians

CRAM SESSION IN

Functional Neuroanatomy

A Handbook for Students & Clinicians

MICHAEL F. NOLAN, PHD, PT
Professor of Basic Science and Director of Assessment
Virginia Tech Carilion School of Medicine
Roanoke, Virginia

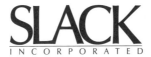

www.slackbooks.com

ISBN: 978-1-61711-009-2

Copyright © 2012 by SLACK Incorporated

Michael F. Nolan has no financial or proprietary interest in the materials presented herein.

The procedures and practices described in this publication should be implemented in a manner consistent with the professional standards set for the circumstances that apply in each specific situation. Every effort has been made to confirm the accuracy of the information presented and to correctly relate generally accepted practices. The authors, editors, and publisher cannot accept responsibility for errors or exclusions or for the outcome of the material presented herein. There is no expressed or implied warranty of this book or information imparted by it. Care has been taken to ensure that drug selection and dosages are in accordance with currently accepted/recommended practice. Off-label uses of drugs may be discussed. Due to continuing research, changes in government policy and regulations, and various effects of drug reactions and interactions, it is recommended that the reader carefully review all materials and literature provided for each drug, especially those that are new or not frequently used. Some drugs or devices in this publication have clearance for use in a restricted research setting by the Food and Drug and Administration or FDA. Each professional should determine the FDA status of any drug or device prior to use in their practice.

SLACK Incorporated uses a review process to evaluate submitted material. Prior to publication, educators or clinicians provide important feedback on the content that we publish. We welcome feedback on this work.

Published by: SLACK Incorporated
                6900 Grove Road
                Thorofare, NJ 08086 USA
                Telephone: 856-848-1000
                Fax: 856-848-6091
                www.slackbooks.com

Contact SLACK Incorporated for more information about other books in this field or about the availability of our books from distributors outside the United States.

Library of Congress Cataloging-in-Publication Data

Nolan, Michael
  Cram session in functional neuroanatomy: a handbook for students & clinicians / Michael F. Nolan.
    p. ; cm. -- (Cram session in physical therapy series)
  Functional neuroanatomy
  Includes bibliographical references and index.
  ISBN 978-1-61711-009-2 (pbk. : alk. paper)
  I. Title. II. Title: Functional neuroanatomy. III. Series: Cram session in physical therapy series.
  [DNLM: 1. Central Nervous System--anatomy & histology--Handbooks. 2. Central Nervous System--physiology--Handbooks. WL 39]

  611'.8--dc23   2011046531

Printed in the United States of America.

Last digit is print number: 10   9   8   7   6   5   4   3   2   1

CONTENTS

ACKNOWLEDGMENTS

The content and organization of this work are the net result of learning and experiential processes that I have been influenced by during my academic career. During that time, different versions of this book have been developed and used for particular groups of students and their particular learning needs. Many students have used this material in their studies and many have offered feedback and suggestions for its improvement. In particular I would like to acknowledge the feedback I received from the physical therapy and medical students of the College of Medicine at the University of South Florida and the first-year medical students of the Virginia Tech Carilion School of Medicine. Their comments were helpful in making sure the text was clear and understandable. In addition, I would like to thank the resident physicians in the departments of Neurology and Neurosurgery at USF for their suggestions and help in making sure that the focus and emphasis of individual chapters remained on clinically relevant concepts and topics. I am certain that I learned as much from them as they did from me.

I must also thank my best friend and wife Debby, who insisted that I continue to revise each chapter until I was satisfied that each was "finally finished" and ready for submission.

Finally, I would like to acknowledge the work of Debra Toulson and her staff at SLACK Incorporated for taking the multiple hard copy and digital parts of this work and turning them into the book you have in your hands.

ABOUT THE AUTHOR

Michael F. Nolan, PhD, PT received a bachelor's degree in physical therapy from Marquette University and a PhD in anatomy (neuroanatomy) from the Medical College of Wisconsin.

Dr. Nolan is Director of Assessment at the Virginia Tech Carilion School of Medicine and Research Institute in Roanoke, Virginia, where he holds the rank of Professor in the Department of Basic Science. He is also Professor Emeritus of Pathology and Cell Biology at the University of South Florida, where he received numerous teaching awards for both undergraduate and graduate medical education, including the John M. Thompson, MD Outstanding Teacher Award in Neurosurgery.

He is the author of *Introduction to the Neurologic Examination* and *Clinical Applications of Human Anatomy.*

INTRODUCTION

Our ability to understand how injury or disease involving the nervous system influences human behavior requires a reasonable understanding of the structure and function of the various, interrelated components of the nervous system. This book is designed to provide the reader with a concise overview of key principles regarding human nervous system structure and function.

The book is organized primarily to facilitate understanding of nervous system function with specific sections dealing with sensory and motor functions, functions mediated by the cranial nerves and the so-called higher cortical functions. Additional sections are included that focus on the gross anatomical organization of the nervous system and the physical environment in which the nervous system is located. These latter sections address such topics as the blood supply and venous drainage of the brain, the multi-layered meningeal coverings of the central nervous system, and the carefully regulated fluid environment both within and surrounding the brain that is necessary for normal nerve cell function.

Each section is composed of chapters that deal with specific topics commonly understood to be important in developing an understanding of that particular nervous system function. Basic information is presented in the form of Key Points related to the subject of each chapter. Feedback regarding one's success in acquiring an understanding of the key points is provided online in the form of short answer Topic Self-Assessment exercises and multiple-choice formatted Practice Exam Questions; questions similar to those that might be encountered on standardized examinations. For learners who favor visual methods or who may be using this book in conjunction with nervous system models, atlases, or actual brain specimens, a list of Laboratory Structures has been included for each chapter online.

The book is intended for students in the health professions who are looking for a concise, clinically-relevant introduction to or review of human neuroanatomy. For students studying functional neuroanatomy for the first time, individual topics are covered in sufficient depth to permit an adequate understanding of the subject, but not in so much detail that valuable time is lost or diverted from other studies or learning activities. Students with a previous academic or clinical background in functional neuroanatomy will find the depth of coverage quite adequate for the purpose of review.

The book is intended for use in both formal and informal learning settings. The arrangement and organization of topics covered in each section might easily serve as the outline for formal courses in functional neuroanatomy within a professional health care curriculum. The book is also effective when used as part of an independent study effort, such as when preparing for a professional certification examination. In the current climate of compressed curricula and increased desire for independent study approaches, this book indeed represents a "cram session in functional neuroanatomy."

Cram Session in Functional Neuroanatomy includes ancillary materials specifically available for faculty use. Included are Practice Exam Questions, Topic Self-Assessments, and Laboratory Structures. Please visit www.efacultylounge.com to obtain access.

SECTION I

Structure and Organization of the Nervous System

Nolan M.
Cram Session in Functional Neuroanatomy:
A Handbook for Students & Clinicians (pp. 1-40)
© 2012 SLACK Incorporated

NEUROCYTOLOGY

Key Points

1. Nerve cells (neurons) develop through a process of cell division involving specialized neuroepithelial cells that form the embryonic neural tube and neural crest. The alar lamina of the neural tube gives rise to association cells (interneurons and long tract cells). The basal lamina of the neural tube gives rise to efferent cells (somatic motor neurons, branchiomeric motor neurons and preganglionic autonomic neurons). The neural crest is the origin of afferent cells, the noradrenergic cells of the adrenal medulla and postganglionic nerve cells of the autonomic nervous system as well as several other cell types not typically considered to be part of the nervous system. Neural structures that form the peripheral nervous system (PNS) are derived from the basal lamina and the neural crest. Most of the cells of the central nervous system (CNS) are derived from the embryonic alar lamina. (Cells located within the CNS with axons that pass out of the CNS as part of a particular cranial nerve or spinal nerve are derived from the basal lamina.)

2. Neurons are morphologically the most diverse cell type in the body. They are also the most complex cell from a biochemical perspective, housing the genetic and metabolic apparatus for synthesizing a wide variety of protein products. Neurons rely almost exclusively on glucose as a substrate for their high-energy requirements.

3. Although neurons as a class are the most diverse cell type of the body in terms of their size and anatomical structure, they essentially are of three fundamental shapes: bipolar, pseudounipolar, and multipolar (Figure 1-1). Bipolar and pseudounipolar cells represent the smallest population quantitatively. These cells are derived from the neural crest and function as afferent cells. They are associated with both the general and special senses. Multipolar cells represent greater than 99.9% of the nerve cells of the CNS and PNS with the vast majority of these arising from the alar and basal lamina of the neural tube. Some multipolar cells are derived from the neural crest. Neural crest-derived multipolar cells migrate to form postganglionic autonomic nerve cells located throughout the body and the cells of the adrenal medulla.

4. The anatomical components of the bipolar cell and the pseudounipolar cell are the cell body and the peripheral and central processes. (*Note*: these cells do not have axons and dendrites in the conventional sense, but rather demonstrate two cytoplasmic processes that extend from

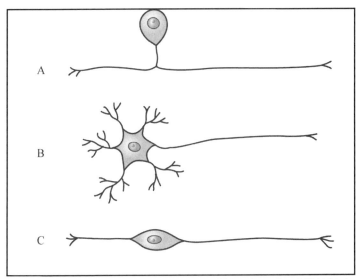

Figure 1-1: Morphologic cell types in the nervous system. (A) Pseudounipolar cell. (B) Multipolar cell. (C) Bipolar cell.

the cell body: the peripheral process, which extends peripherally from the cell body, and the central process, which extends centrally from the cell body.)

5. Bipolar cells bodies are found in the retina, where they are associated with the optic nerve and the visual system, and in the vestibular and cochlear ganglia, where they are associated with the vestibular and cochlear nerves, respectively. In bipolar cells associated with the vestibular and cochlear nerves, the peripheral process is the shorter of the two cellular processes. The distal end of the peripheral process makes synaptic contact with specialized receptor cells (hair cells) found in the inner ear (see further discussion in sections dealing with the vestibular and auditory systems.) Nerve impulses are transmitted toward the cell body (centripetally) along the peripheral process. Intra-axonal transport is bidirectional in the peripheral process. The central process is the longer of the two cellular processes. This process is myelinated extends toward the CNS, contributing to the vestibular or cochlear nerve. The central process enters the CNS and terminates by making synaptic contact with cells that form either the vestibular or cochlear nuclei. Nerve impulses are transmitted away from the cell body (centrifugally) along the central process.

6. Pseudounipolar cells are located in dorsal root ganglia and in selected sensory ganglia associated with certain cranial nerves. The peripheral process of a pseudounipolar cell is the longer of the two cell processes and may be myelinated or unmyelinated. The distal end of the peripheral process may end as a free nerve ending or may make synaptic contact with a receptor (sensory transducer). Nerve impulses are transmitted toward the cell body along the peripheral process. The central process is the shorter of the two processes. Those associated with cranial nerves enter the brainstem and terminate in various nuclei within the brainstem. Those associated with spinal nerves form dorsal roots and terminate either in the spinal cord or in the caudal part of the medulla oblongata. The central process is myelinated. The region of the central process closest to the cell body is myelinated by Schwann cells, while the region closest to the CNS is myelinated by oligodendrocytes. The point along the length of the central process that marks the change in myelin-producing cells is referred to as the Obersteiner-Redlich line. Nerve impulses are transmitted away from the cell body along the central process.

7. The anatomical components of the multipolar neuron are the cell body (soma, perikaryon), dendrites, axon, and synaptic ending. Each has its own specialized morphology and function.

8. The cell body is the location of the nucleus of the cell and the location of protein synthesis within the cell. A variety of proteins are synthesized by neurons including membrane proteins, cytoskeletal proteins, secretory proteins, and enzymes.

9. Dendrites are cytoplasmic extensions of the cell body, functioning as the "receptive" part of the cell. The dendritic cell membrane is characterized by the presence of receptor proteins, ion channel proteins, and the absence of a myelin sheath. Some dendrites demonstrate smooth surfaces while others are characterized by small dendritic "spines." Dendrites do not propagate action potentials.

10. Axons are cytoplasmic extensions, the membrane of which is characterized by the presence of ion channels, and in some instances, a covering by myelin. Axons in the PNS can be myelinated or unmyelinated. Myelin in the PNS is produced by Schwann cells. Axons in the CNS are myelinated. In the CNS, myelin is produced by oligodendrocytes. Axons typically contain a variety of intracellular structures including microfilaments, neurofilaments, and neurotubules. Microfilaments (5 nm) are formed by actin monomers and are present in growth cones. Neurofilaments (10 nm) are associated with tau proteins. Neurotubules (20 to 30 nm) are important structures in the processes of anterograde and retrograde axonal transport.

11. Axons typically branch at their distal end, giving rise to collateral branches. Axons transmit "information" by means of nerve impulses, so-called electrical transmission, and by way of intra-axonal transport mechanisms along intracellular cytoskeletal elements, specifically neurotubules. Intracellular transport mechanisms move substances bidirectionally along the outer surface of microtubules within the axon. Orthograde transport (away from the cell body) is powered by kinesin molecules and occurs at two speeds. Rapid orthograde transport (200 to 300 mm/day) carries membrane proteins, transmitter proteins, and amino acids. Slow orthograde transport (0.2 to 5 mm/day) carries cytoskeletal proteins and metabolic enzymes. Retrograde transport (toward the cell body) is powered by dynein molecules and occurs rapidly (150 to 200 mm/day). Substances transported toward the cell body include toxins, viruses, and growth factors.

12. The synaptic ending (synaptic bouton) is located at the distal extent of the axon. The synaptic ending together with the postsynaptic membrane and the intervening space (synaptic cleft) constitute the *synapse*. Neurotransmitters are released from the synaptic ending by a process of exocytosis. Some neurotransmitters are synthesized in the synaptic ending and others are synthesized in the cell body and transported to the synaptic ending. Transmitter substances released from the presynaptic membrane diffuse into the synaptic cleft and bind to receptor proteins embedded in the membrane of the postsynaptic cell, resulting in the movement of ions across the postsynaptic cell membrane and changes in the behavior of that cell. Fundamentally, neurotransmitters act to either excite or inhibit the postsynaptic cell. Compounds known to function as neurotransmitters include amino acids (glutamate, glycine, GABA, aspartate), biogenic amines (NE, DA, 5HT, histamine), neuropeptides (SP, ENK, VIP, NPY, oxytocin, somatostatin), and acetylcholine. Receptor proteins of the postsynaptic membrane are of two fundamental types: ionotropic receptors and metabotropic receptors.

13. Nerve cell membranes are unique in that their structure includes a large number of proteins. Nerve cell membranes are particularly rich in alpha helix proteins in the form of receptors and globular proteins in the form of ion channels. Energy is required to maintain the structure and function of the membrane and the membrane-associated proteins. For example, failure to provide the energy necessary to operate the "ion pumps" located in nerve cell membranes results in the diffusion of ions down their concentration gradients and a loss of the functionally essential membrane potential. In such cases, potassium will move out of the cell and sodium and chloride will move into the

Table 1-1

Classification of Neurons

Function—Afferent, efferent, association (interneurons)
Effect—Excitatory, inhibitory
Morphology—Multipolar, bipolar, pseudounipolar
Shape—Mitral, basket, granule, stellate, pyramidal
Location—Ganglia, nucleus, cortex
Neurotransmitter—Cholinergic, glutamatergic, adrenergic, GABAergic
Eponym—Purkinje, Renshaw, Cajal, Golgi, Betz, Waldeyer
Axon Length—Golgi I (long), Golgi II (short)
Embryonic Origin—Neural crest, alar lamina, basal lamina

cell along with water. The result will be cellular swelling (cytotoxic edema) and possibly death of the cell.

14. Neurons are constantly dying throughout both the prenatal and post-natal life of the individual. Some cells die as a consequence of injury through a process known as *necrosis*. Others die for reasons that are genetically controlled by mechanisms of programmed cell death, one type of which is known as *apoptosis* (Table 1-1).

NEUROGLIA

Key Points

1. The major cell types of the CNS (brain and spinal cord) are nerve cells (neurons) and neuroglia. Neuroglia (glia or glial cells for short) are of two types: macroglia and microglia. Macroglia include astrocytes (protoplasmic and fibrous) and oligodendrocytes (oligodendroglia or "oligos" for short). Microglia include microglial cells. Glial cells constitute 50% of the brain by volume but represent 90% of the cells that form the brain. The glial cell to nerve cell ratio is calculated to be 9:1.

2. Astrocytes and oligodendroglia, like nerve cells, are embryologically derived from neuroectoderm. Microglia are derived from blood-borne monocytes that migrate into the developing CNS before closure of the blood-brain barrier.

3. Astrocytes constitute approximately 15% of the brain by volume and represent approximately 35% to 40% of the glial cell population.

Astrocytes are stellate shaped cells with small cell bodies and a prominent nucleus. These cells have relatively little cytoplasm and are generally distinguished by their nuclear characteristics. Protoplasmic astrocytes are found predominantly in gray matter and fibrous astrocytes are located predominantly in white matter. Morphologically, astrocytes may be difficult to distinguish from small neurons (although astrocytes may have multiple nucleoli). Chemically, astrocytes, unlike neurons, are marked by glial fibrillary acidic protein (GFAP), an intermediate filament and the main cytoskeletal element of the cell. GFAP is easily stained in histological preparations. Astrocytes, like neurons, have membrane receptors for many neurotransmitters and neuropeptides as well as both voltage-gated and ligand-gated ion channels (although astrocytes do not generate action potentials). Astrocytes, like neurons, require energy to maintain their function. Energy failure in astrocytes can lead to such outcomes such as cell swelling (a cytotoxic form of edema) and possible neuronal excitotoxicity from the release of glutamate into the extracellular environment. Importantly, astrocytes have membrane uptake mechanisms for amino acid (glutamate and GABA) and monoamine neurotransmitters.

4. When first discovered, astrocytes were thought to function as a type of glue or connective substance that held nerve cells together, providing only structural support for the nervous system. (The word *glia* is derived from the word "Nervenkitt" meaning "nerve glue.") Astrocytes were often referred to as "supporting" cells, implying nothing more than anatomical or structural support. Astrocytes are indeed supportive, but support is now understood to include metabolic, physiologic, and functional support as well as structural support.

5. The major functions/roles of astrocytes are listed below:

    a. Define the limit (boundary/extent) of the CNS

    b. Induce formation of the blood-brain barrier

    c. Function as a buffer for ionic movement in the CNS

    d. Participate in neurotransmitter regulation (glutamine shuttle)

    e. Participate in glucose/glycogen metabolism

    f. Guide neuronal migration during development

    g. React to injury (trauma, toxins)

h. Involvement in and responses to disease conditions and processes

i. Aid in neuronal and nervous system repair

6. a. Near the surface of the brain, astrocyte foot processes make direct contact with pial cells forming the glia-pial membrane (glia limitans). The glia limitans effectively and completely envelopes the brain such that nerve cells do not directly come into contact with any cells other that astrocytes. The glia limitans serves to "internalize" the brain and to define the anatomical boundary of the CNS.

7. b. During development, astrocytes make anatomical contact with the invading and developing vasculature of the brain. Astrocytic contact induces the formation of tight junctions between endothelial cells, thereby promoting development of the functional structure referred to as the blood-brain-barrier (BBB). (Only in certain areas of the brain, namely the majority of the circumventricular organs, is the BBB absent.) In the mature (adult) nervous system, astrocyte foot processes wrap around brain capillaries, thereby both insulating nerve cells from direct contact with these non-ectodermal-derived cells and facilitating mechanisms whereby substances taken up by the brain pass initially through or are processed by astrocytes.

8. c. Membrane mechanisms in astrocytes can take up K+ from the extracellular space of the brain as occurs when neurons are normally active or excessively active as is the case in certain abnormal conditions. Excess intracellular K+ can be transported into the vascular system or distributed to other astrocytes in the neighborhood by means of direct cell to cell connections (gap junctions) between astrocytes. This buffering mechanism functions to help stabilize and normalize ionic concentrations of potassium in the extracellular fluid (ECF). This mechanism may be particularly important in the brain's response to seizure activity.

9. d. Astrocyte foot processes are found in close proximity to synaptic endings and participate in synaptic events, particularly in the inactivation of glutamate (GLU) and GABA (95% of the synapses in the brain use either GLU or GABA). With regard to GLU, after acting on glutamate receptors, GLU is taken up by nearby astrocytes and there converted into glutamine (by glutamine synthetase). Glutamine is then transported back into the nerve cell to be converted again into GLU—a process sometimes referred to as the *glutamine shuttle*. (Glutamine synthetase is found exclusively in astrocytes.)

10. e. The brain utilizes glucose almost exclusively as an energy source, and in fact, utilizes 20% of the glucose transported in the blood-

stream. Two mechanisms for glucose utilization by the brain have been described. In one, sometimes referred to as the *preferred pathway*, glucose is transported from the bloodstream into astrocytes, where it is converted into glycogen (in small quantities for brief storage) or pyruvate and then to lactate. (Some pyruvate is used to make ATP for use as energy by the astrocyte.) Lactate produced in astrocytes is then transported into neurons, where it is used to make pyruvate and then ATP (fuel for the nerve cell). In the other, sometimes referred to as the *alternate pathway*, nerve cells take up glucose directly to be converted into pyruvate and then ATP.

11. f. During the early stages of nervous system development, some glial cells play a special role in the migration of nerve cells from the proliferative zone of the primitive neural tube to their definitive location either deep within the brain, where they form nuclei, or to the surface of the brain, where they form the cortices of the cerebrum or cerebellum. These specialized glial cells, referred to as *radial glia*, essentially function as a scaffold along which nerve cells migrate to their predetermined, final location. A similar function in the cerebellum is performed by Bergman glia.

12. g. Astrocytes play an important role in the response to injury involving the nervous system. In cases of trauma, glial cells may undergo hypertrophy and hyperplasia (reactive gliosis), resulting in the formation of glial scars. Such scars may impede neuronal regeneration or serve as a focus of seizure activity. Glial cells responding to injury demonstrate significant increases in GFAP.

13. h. Astrocytes play an important role in the response to various disease processes affecting the nervous system. For example, with infection of the nervous system, glial cells become activated, proliferate, and "wall off" the infection. A similar response may be seen with certain types of metastatic neoplasia (cancer). Most brain tumors are composed of glial cells (astrocytomas and oligodendrogliomas). Disease processes that impair astrocyte function may lead to glial release of glutamate, which may in turn lead to excitotoxicity and functional impairment. Hepatic encephalopathy results when excess ammonia resulting from liver disease impairs astrocyte ability to clear glutamate released from nerve cells. Excessive glutamate results in excitotoxicity, which in turn results in nerve cell and brain dysfunction manifested as confusion, seizures, or coma. Glial cells are also affected by brain ischemia (stroke). Ischemia affecting astrocytes can result in reversal of ion transport mechanisms, one of which (Na+) is coupled to the movement of glutamate. Reperfusion after stroke can result in movement of both Na+ and glutamate out of astrocytes and

the subsequent development of excitotoxicity, particularly in the area of the ischemic penumbra.

14. i. Astrocytes release molecules that facilitate repair after injury. Some molecules break down the extracellular matrix to permit synaptic reorganization, while others lay down extracellular matrix to help stabilize synaptic structures. Astrocytes also release various cell adhesion molecules.

15. Oligodendroglia are the myelin-producing cells of the CNS and are arguably the most distinctive and strangely shaped cells in the body! Oligodendroglia are of two types: fascicular oligodendrocytes, located in the white matter of the brain, and perineuronal oligodendrocytes, found in the gray matter.

16. Myelin is formed by multiple layers of the cell membrane of an oligodendroglial cell wrapped tightly around a segment of an axon. Myelin is up to 80% lipid, with cholesterol and cerebroside accounting for approximately 50% of the lipid content. In the CNS, a single oligodendroglial cell provides segmental myelin for several (up to 40) nearby axons (unlike in the PNS, where Schwann cells produce myelin for only a single segment of a single axon). Gaps between myelin segments in the CNS are known as *nodes of Ranvier* (just as they are in the PNS).

17. The process of myelination in the CNS is incomplete at birth and continues during the first two decades of life. This may account for the poor motor function observed in newborns and toddlers.

18. Lesions affecting axons in the CNS result in anterograde axonal degeneration similar to that seen in the PNS. However, anatomical regeneration in the CNS does not occur (at least to date) partly as a result of several factors, including the absence of connective tissue structures to guide axonal regeneration and to the presence of certain proteins such as Nogo, which prevent the development of growth cones.

19. Certain diseases, such as multiple sclerosis, affect oligodendrocytes in small, circumscribed areas resulting in focal areas of demyelination (plaques). Neuronal function is impaired or lost, with the signs and symptoms reflecting the functional neural systems affected.

20. Microglia are frequently considered to be the resident macrophage of the nervous system and the major representative of the immune system in the brain. Microglia are not ectodermal derived cells, but rather enter the nervous system early during development, when the BBB is not yet formed. They remain quiet in the brain until activated by injury or infection.

21. Microglia are active in two circumstances: during the embryonic period and in response to injury or infection. During the embryonic period, microglia remove debris associated with the process of programmed cell death. In the mature nervous system, in the presence of injury or infection, microglia enter the "activated" state. When activated, microglia increase in size, withdraw their cytoplasmic processes, become ameboid, and migrate to the site of infection where they become phagocytic. Activated microglia secrete cytokines and can become antigen-presenting cells. Some evidence suggests that excessive microglial activity can result in damage to neurons.

GROSS BRAIN AND BRAINSTEM

Key Points

1. The CNS is defined as the brain and spinal cord. The brain is composed of the forebrain, brainstem, and cerebellum. The structures of the CNS are formed by nerve cells (neurons) and glial cells derived largely from the embryonic neural tube. During development, neuroblasts and glioblasts, the result of mitotic activity in the embryonic neural tube, migrate away from the lumen of the neural tube for varying distances toward the developing meninges. The result of these mitotic and migratory processes will be the development and placement of populations of neurons and glial cells in specific locations between the deepest layer of the meninges (pia mater) and the ependymal lining of the neural lumen. These cells and their processes (axons and dendrites) form the differentially thick wall of the neural tube and constitute the largest portion of the CNS.

2. The rate of cell division is different in different regions of the neural tube. This results in an uneven distribution of cells in different regions of the developing neural tube and gives rise to the peculiar shape and histologic organization of the forebrain and brainstem. In the forebrain, nerve cell bodies located immediately deep to the meningeal layer near the surface of the developing brain form the cerebral cortex. Cell bodies located more deeply within the hemisphere form nuclei such as the lenticular nuclei, the amygdaloid nuclei, and the nuclei of the thalamus. Located between the cell bodies that form the cerebral cortex and those that form the more deeply located nuclei is a region composed of myelinated axonal processes. Grossly, areas consisting predominantly of nerve cell bodies (cortex and nuclei) are referred to a gray matter while areas consisting primarily of myelinated axons are referred to as white matter.

3. The brain is commonly divided into distinct anatomical regions or parts using one of several classification schemes. Some classification methods are based on embryological concepts (ie, telencephalon, diencephalon, mesencephalon, metencephalon, and myelencephalon) while others are based on the gross anatomical principles (ie, forebrain, brainstem, and cerebellum). Not infrequently, terms from several classification systems are used together when describing brain structure and organization. The brief descriptions below borrow from these multiple systems.

4. The forebrain is composed of structures derived from the telencephalon and diencephalon. Telencephalon-derived structures include the cerebral cortex and most of the basal nuclei. These structures comprise the largest part of the cerebral hemisphere. Each cerebral hemisphere is commonly subdivided into lobes (frontal, parietal, occipital, and temporal), each of which plays a major role in particular neurologic functions. Each lobe consists of four components: a cortical layer, a collection of nerve cell bodies that form deep nuclei, a region of intervening white matter, and a portion of the ventricular system. The cortical layer consists of a thin layer of cells located immediately deep to the innermost layer of the meninges. This cell layer is organized into folds resulting in surface elevations (convolutions) referred to as *gyri* and grooves or infoldings referred to as *sulci* or *fissures*. The major nuclei of the telencephalic portion of the forebrain include the caudate, putamen, and amygdala. The intervening white matter (subcortical white) consists of axons that transmit nerve impulses to and from the cells of the cerebral cortex (projection fibers), to and from the cells located within a hemisphere (association fibers), and to and from cells located in the opposite hemisphere (commissural fibers). These axons are frequently grouped and named in relation to a particular functional system of which they are a part. Each hemisphere also contains a portion of the ventricular system, the adult remnant of the embryonic neural tube. The right and left lateral ventricles are located within the substance of each telencephalic hemisphere (Figures 1-2 and 1-3).

5. The diencephalon is composed of the dorsal thalamus (commonly referred to simply as the *thalamus*), hypothalamus, ventral thalamus, epithalamus and subthalamus. The dorsal thalamus is formed by groups of nuclei, most of which relay information to the cerebral cortex. Some nuclei give rise to specific projections to restricted areas of the cortex, while others are characterized by a widespread cortical distribution. The hypothalamus consists of small, tightly packed nuclei that influence predominantly the pituitary gland and

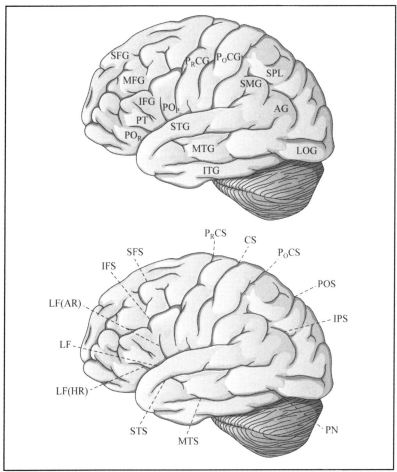

Figure 1-2: Cerebral gyri and sulci of the lateral surface of the hemisphere. *Key for gyri*: SFG=superior frontal gyrus, MFG=middle frontal gyrus, IFG=inferior frontal gyrus, PO$_R$=pars orbitalis, PT=pars triangularis, PO$_P$=pars opercularis, P$_R$CG=precentral gyrus, P$_O$CG=postcentral gyrus, SPL=superior parietal lobule, SMG=supramarginal gyrus, AG=angular gyrus, LOG=lateral occipital gyrus, STG=superior temporal gyrus, MTG=middle temporal gyrus, ITG=inferior temporal gyrus. *Key for sulci*: LF (HR)=lateral fissure (horizontal ramus), LF=lateral fissure (sylvian), LF (AR)=lateral fissure (ascending ramus), IFS=inferior frontal sulcus, SFS=superior frontal sulcus, P$_R$CS=precentral sulcus, CS=central sulcus (rolandic), P$_O$CS=postcentral sulcus, POS=parietooccipital sulcus, IPS=intraparietal sulcus, PN=preoccipital notch, MTS=middle temporal sulcus, STS=superior temporal sulcus.

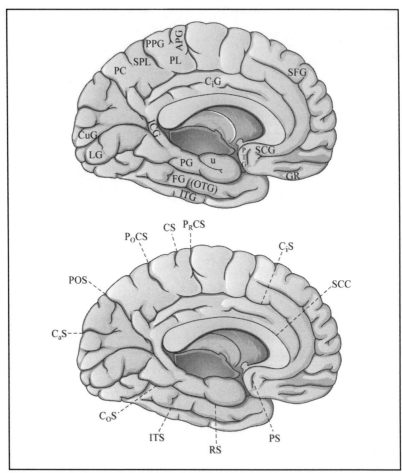

Figure 1-3: Cerebral gyri and sulci of the medial surface of the hemisphere. *Key for gyri*: SFG=superior frontal gyrus, ITG=inferior temporal gyrus, C$_u$G=cuneate gyrus, LG=lingual gyrus, PC=precuneus, PL=paracentral lobule, PPG=posterior paracentral gyrus, APG=anterior paracentral gyrus, C$_i$G=cingulate gyrus, ICG=isthmus of the cingulate gyrus, U=uncus, PG=parahippocampal gyrus, FG=fusiform gyrus (occipito-temporal gyrus), PTG=paraterminal gyrus, SCG=subcallosal gyrus, GR=gyrus rectus. *Key for sulci*: P$_R$CS=precentral sulcus, CS=central sulcus (rolandic), P$_O$CS=postcentral sulcus, POS=parietooccipital sulcus, C$_a$S=calcarine sulcus, C$_i$S=cingulate sulcus, SCC=sulcus of the corpus callosum, PS=paraterminal sulcus, RS=rhinal sulcus, ITS=inferior temporal sulcus, C$_O$S=collateral sulcus.

cells of the autonomic nervous system. The ventral thalamus consists of the subthalamic nucleus, zona incerta, and the pre-rubral fields (of Forel). The epithalamus is formed by the pineal gland, habenular nuclei and commissure, and the posterior commissure. The metathalamic nuclei include the lateral and medial geniculate nuclei, and relay nuclei in the visual and auditory systems. The third ventricle, located in the midline between the two halves of the dorsal thalamus and hypothalamus, is the adult remnant of the lumen of the embryonic neural tube at the level of the diencephalon.

6. The brainstem consists of three parts extending caudally from the forebrain to the spinal cord. These parts are the midbrain, pons, and medulla oblongata, derived from the embryonic mesencephalon, metencephalon, and myelencephalon, respectively. The brainstem is considerably smaller than the forebrain in size, suggesting that considerably less cell division and migration occurred at these segmental levels during embryogenesis. The brainstem consists of nerve cell bodies forming nuclei, axons forming fiber tracts and a portion of the ventricular system. (Unlike the forebrain, the brainstem does not demonstrate a superficial, cortical layer of cells.) The nuclei of the brainstem are of two general types: those that contain either efferent or association cell bodies. Efferent cells are associated with axons that are part of certain cranial nerves. Association cells are the origin of axons that either form local circuits within the brainstem or contribute to pathways that project to nerve cells outside the brainstem in the forebrain, cerebellum, or spinal cord. The fiber tracts of the brainstem are also of two general types: those that simply pass through the brainstem, arising and terminating in other parts of the nervous system, and those that originate or terminate within in the brainstem, thereby connecting the brainstem with cells in the forebrain, cerebellum, or spinal cord. The components of the ventricular system found in the brainstem include the cerebral aqueduct (of Sylvius) located in the midbrain and the fourth ventricle located in the pons and rostral part of the medulla oblongata.

7. The cerebellum occupies the posterior cranial fossa (infratentorial compartment) together with the brainstem. It is separated from the occipital lobe by the tentorium cerebelli. The cerebellum consists of two large hemispheres separated by a small midline portion, the vermis. Grossly, the cerebellum is divided into three lobes: the flocculonodular lobe, the anterior lobe, and the posterior lobe. The terms *archicerebellum, paleocerebellum,* and *neocerebellum,* used to describe the cerebellum from a phylogenetic or developmental perspective, are sometimes used to refer to the flocculonodular lobe, anterior lobe,

and posterior lobe, respectively. The cerebellum is attached to the brainstem by three bundles of axons: the superior, middle, and inferior cerebellar peduncles. The superior cerebellar peduncle (brachium conjunctivum) is attached at the level of the midbrain and connects the cerebellum with cells primarily in the midbrain and thalamus. The middle cerebellar peduncle (brachium pontis) is attached at the level of the pons and is formed by axons that transmit impulses from the pons to the cerebellum. The inferior cerebellar peduncle (restiform and juxtarestiform bodies) is connected at the level of the medulla oblongata. The inferior cerebellar peduncle transmits information principally to the cerebellum from cells in the spinal cord and medulla oblongata.

8. The structure of the cerebellum is similar to that of the cerebral cortex in that the cerebellum is characterized by a cortical layer, a collection of deep nuclei, and an intervening layer of axons. The cortex of the cerebellum, like the cortex of the cerebrum, is thrown into folds; however, the folds are smaller and referred to as *folia*. However, unlike the cerebral cortex, the cerebellar cortex demonstrates a consistent three-layered histological organization. The deep nuclei of the cerebellum include the fastigial, globosus, emboliform, and dentate. These cells are the main source of axons that pass out of the cerebellum by way of the cerebellar peduncles.

THALAMUS

Key Points

1. The term *thalamus*, as commonly used, refers to a specific group of nuclei situated deep within the cerebral hemisphere. The thalamus, or more properly the dorsal thalamus, is one of five anatomical divisions of the diencephalon. These five diencephalic components are the dorsal thalamus, hypothalamus, ventral thalamus (subthalamic nucleus, zona incerta, and the fields of Forel), epithalamus (pituitary gland, habenular nuclei, and the posterior commissure), and metathalamus (medial and lateral geniculate nuclei). Most diencephalic structures are paired, being located on either side of the third ventricle.

2. Most of the nuclei that make up the dorsal thalamus are relay nuclei composed of cells with axons that project to and terminate in the cerebral cortex. One nucleus (central medial) is formed by cells that project axons to the striatum; another (reticular nucleus) is the origin of projections to other dorsal thalamic nuclei. Some nuclei give rise to axons that project to comparatively small, circumscribed cortical

areas while others are the origin of projections that terminate widely throughout the cerebral cortex. Some nuclei are part of specific functional systems (sensory, motor, visual, auditory, cognitive and emotional), while others are part of systems that are not clearly part of specific experiential or behavioral systems.

3. The dorsal thalamus, the largest of the five components of the diencephalon, is composed of two egg-shaped collections of nuclei bounded superiorly by the floor of the lateral ventricle; medially by the third ventricle; and anteriorly, ventrally, and laterally by the internal capsule. Caudally, the thalamus merges with the rostral part of the midbrain with the traditional boundary described as being a line extending inferiorly from the posterior edge of the posterior commissure to the posterior edge of the mammillary body.

4. The nuclei that comprise the dorsal thalamus are classically described as forming several groups. These groups include the lateral group (which includes a ventral tier and dorsal tier), the medial group, the anterior group, the intralaminar group, the reticular group, and the midline group.

5. The lateral nuclear group is located lateral to the internal medullary lamina (of the thalamus) and medial to the external medullary lamina (of the thalamus). The anterior part of this group is separated from the anterior group by the lateral arm of the internal medullary lamina. The ventral tier nuclei include ventral anterior (VA), ventral lateral (VL), ventral medial (VM), and the ventral posterior nuclei, which include ventral posterior lateral (VPL) and ventral posterior medial (VPM). These nuclei are sometimes referred to as "relay" nuclei since they essentially relay nerve impulses from specific nuclei of the spinal cord, brainstem, and diencephalon to specific, relatively focal areas of the cerebral cortex. The dorsal tier nuclei include lateral dorsal (LD), lateral posterior (LP), and the pulvinar (P). These nuclei are the origin of axonal projections that terminate rather more diffusely in the cerebral cortex.

6. The major afferent and efferent connections of the above listed dorsal thalamic, lateral group nuclei will be briefly summarized below. VA receives input from the globus pallidus (ipsilateral) and projects to the premotor and supplementary motor cortices. VL receives input from the cerebellum (contralateral) and red nucleus (ipsilateral) and projects to the primary motor cortex (precentral gyrus and anterior paracentral gyrus). VM lies ventral and medial to the VA/VL groups and likely receives convergent projections from the ipsilateral globus pallidus, contralateral cerebellum, and ipsilateral red nucleus. Projections from VM likely terminate in the premotor, supplementary

motor, and primary motor cortices. VPL receives input from the dorsal column nuclei (contralateral) by way of the medial lemniscus and the spinal cord (contralateral) by way of the spinal lemniscus and projects to the body areas of the primary somatosensory cortex (postcentral gyrus and posterior paracentral gyrus). VPM receives input from the spinal nucleus of the trigeminal nerve (contralateral) by way of the ventral trigeminothalamic tract and the principal nucleus of the trigeminal nerve (bilateral) by way of the dorsal trigeminothalamic tracts, and projects to the face area of the postcentral gyrus. LD and LP are small nuclei of the dorsal tier that are reciprocally connected with the cingulate gyrus and parietal lobe, respectively. The pulvinar receives input from the superior colliculus and projects axons to the visual association cortex of the occipital lobe. Other projections arising from the pulvinar, thought to be involved in aspects of visual and ocular motor function, terminate in the frontal lobe.

7. The medial group is located lateral to the third ventricle and medial to the internal medullary lamina. The anterior part of this group is separated from the anterior nuclear group by the medial arm of the internal medullary lamina. The medial nuclear group consists primarily of the dorsal medial nucleus (DM). DM receives input from the spinal cord and the amygdaloid nucleus and projects to the prefrontal cortices including the anterior regions of the cingulate gyrus.

8. The anterior group (A) is located dorsally and anteriorly within the dorsal thalamus, between the medial and lateral arms of the internal medullary lamina. The anterior nucleus receives input from the mammillary nucleus of the hypothalamus and projects to the cingulate gyrus. The axons of the mamillothalamic tract lie within the internal medullary lamina. The axons of this tract, together with the mammillary nucleus and anterior thalamic nucleus, are part of the Papez circuit, an important pathway of the limbic system.

9. The intralaminar group (IL) is located within the thin sheet of fibers that forms the posterior region of the internal medullary lamina. The intralaminar group includes the central median (CM), parafascicular (Pf), and central lateral (CL) nuclei. CM receives input from the globus pallidus and projects to the striatum and to the motor cortices of the frontal lobe. Input to Pf and CL are incompletely understood but is thought to include the spinal cord. Projections from these nuclei are also not well understood but are believed to include association cortices of the frontal and parietal lobes.

10. The reticular nucleus consists of a thin sheet of cells situated on the lateral aspect of the dorsal thalamus, located between the external medullary lamina and the posterior limb of the internal capsule. The cells of the reticular nucleus receive input from the cerebral

cortex (collateral branches of corticothalamic projections) and from the dorsal thalamus (collateral branches of thalamocortical projections). Reticular nucleus cells project widely to cells in all regions of the dorsal thalamus. Unlike most cells of the dorsal thalamus, which synthesize and release excitatory transmitters, the cells of the reticular nucleus release GABA, an inhibitory transmitter. Thus, the reticular nucleus appears to play an important role in modulating the activity of the cells of the dorsal thalamus, thereby influencing the nature of the input to the cortex from the thalamus.

11. The arterial blood supply to the dorsal thalamus is provided by thalamotuberal branches of the posterior communicating artery and the thalamoperforating and thalamogeniculate branches of the posterior cerebral artery. Additional blood supply is provided by penetrating branches of the anterior and posterior choroidal arteries.

SPINAL CORD

Key Points

1. The spinal cord, together with the forebrain and brainstem, constitute the CNS. In the adult human, the spinal cord extends from the inferior extent of the decussation of the pyramid (approximately at the level of the foramen magnum) to the tip of the conus medullaris (approximately at the level of the L1-L2 intervertebral disk) and is approximately 40 cm in length. (In the neonate and infant, the spinal cord extends caudally to lower lumbar levels. The apparent rise in the level of the tip of the conus medullaris is the result of the relatively greater increase in the length of the vertebral column.)

2. The spinal cord is not uniformly cylindrical throughout its length, but is rather characterized by two "enlargements" involving those spinal segments that provide afferent and efferent innervation to the upper limb (C5-T1) and the lower limb (L2-S2). At these enlarged segments, particularly those associated with the upper limb, the spinal cord is slightly larger from side to side (9 to 14 mm) than from anterior to posterior (6 to 7 mm). At nonlimb segments, the spinal cord demonstrates a more circular structure at the lower ranges of the diameters listed above.

3. The surface of the spinal cord presents several longitudinal grooves running vertically along the length of the cord. The posterior median (dorsal median) fissure is located in the sagittal plane on the posterior (dorsal) surface and extends the full length of the cord. This fissure marks the position of the posterior medial septum. The posterolateral

(dorsolateral) sulcus is located on the posterolateral (dorsolateral) surface of the cord and marks the point of attachment of the dorsal rootlets. The posterolateral sulcus extends the full length of the cord. The posterior intermediate (dorsal intermediate) sulcus lies between the posterior median and posterolateral sulci and marks the position of the posterior intermediate septum. The posterior intermediate sulcus is clearly visible only at cervical spinal cord levels. The anterior median fissure is located in the sagittal plane on the anterior (ventral) surface of the spinal cord. The fissure marks a deep groove in which the linea splendens is located, a thickened sheet of the arachnoid mater together with segmental branches of the anterior spinal artery.

4. The spinal cord is anatomically and functionally divided into longitudinally arranged segments, with a spinal segment being defined as that region (length) of the spinal cord that 1) contains the efferent cell bodies that give rise to axons that form part of a single spinal nerve, and 2) marks the region of attachment of the dorsal rootlets of a single, corresponding spinal nerve. In humans there are 8 cervical, 12 thoracic, 5 lumbar, and 5 sacral spinal segments. Spinal segments range from 8 to 16 mm in length. Spinal segments associated with the brachial and lumbosacral plexuses are larger that those not associated with the innervation of the limbs. Each spinal cord segment is associated with approximately 6 to 8 dorsal and ventral rootlets per segment.

5. The histological organization of the spinal cord is characterized by a central, H-shaped region composed predominantly of nerve cell bodies and their dendrites together with astrocytes (gray matter) surrounded by a region composed primarily of axons and oligodendrocytes (white matter). The gray matter is organized into a dorsal horn, ventral horn, and an intermediate area between the two that includes a small region of central gray surrounding the rudimentary central canal of the cord. A small group of cell bodies located immediately lateral to the intermediate region at spinal levels T1-L2 is sometimes referred to as the *lateral horn*. The number of cells that comprise the gray matter (dorsal and ventral horns and intermediate gray) of spinal segments that form the brachial plexus enlargement and the lumbosacral plexus enlargement is considerably greater than the number found in segments not associated with the innervation of the limbs.

6. The white matter of the spinal cord is organized into a posterior (dorsal) funiculus, lateral funiculus, and anterior (ventral) funiculus. The posterior funiculus is situated between the dorsal horns and extends the full length of the spinal cord. The posterior funiculus is divided into a more medial region, the fasciculus gracilis, which is present at

all levels of the cord and a more lateral region, the fasciculus cuneatus, which is clearly visible only at cervical levels. (The posterior intermediate sulcus is commonly used as a surface landmark marking the boundary between the fasciculus gracilis and cuneatus.) The number of axons in the posterior funiculus at each segment is greater than the number in the segment immediately below. The lateral funiculus is situated laterally, between the dorsal horn and ventral horn. The lateral funiculus is frequently subdivided into a dorsolateral region and a ventrolateral region. The number of axons in the lateral funiculus at each segment is greater than the number in the segment immediately below. The anterior funiculus is situated between the ventral horns and extends the full length of the spinal cord. The anterior funiculus on each side is separated by the anterior median sulcus. The number of axons in the anterior funiculus at each segment is greater than the number in the segment immediately below. Located at the junction of the posterior and lateral funiculi, in a region sometimes referred to as the dorsal root entry zone (DREZ), is a small bundle of axons known as the dorsolateral fasciculus (Lissauer's tract). Lissauer's tract is composed of the ascending and descending central processes of dorsal root ganglion cells (afferent cells) whose peripheral processes are unmyelinated or thinly myelinated. Lissauer's tract also includes a small number of axons of intersegmental interneurons.

7. The white matter of the spinal cord is composed of the axons transmitting nerve impulses either rostrally (to higher levels of the spinal cord or to the brain) or caudally (to lower levels of the spinal cord or from the brain). Most axons are anatomically organized into bundles referred to as *tracts* or *fasciculi*.

8. The spinal cord, like the brain, is enclosed within three layers of the meninges. The dura mater of the spinal cord is the caudal extension of the dura surrounding the brain. However, unlike the dura mater in the cranium, the spinal dura is not adherent to the inner surface of the vertebral column. The spinal dura is separated from the vertebral canal by a space (epidural space) that contains fat and the epidural plexus of veins (Batson's plexus). The spinal dura extends as a sac caudally to the level of the S2 segment of the sacrum where it closes and forms the filum terminale externum, a component of the coccygeal ligament. The arachnoid layer surrounding the spinal cord is continuous caudally with the arachnoid layer surrounding the brain. It lies in close contact with the inner layer of the spinal dura, and like the dura, continues as a sac to the S2 segment of the sacrum, where it too closes, forming the inferior extent of the lumbar cistern. The pia mater of the cord is continuous caudally with the pia surrounding the brain. This

thin layer of the meninges tightly invests the spinal cord, fusing at the tip of the conus medullaris. A thin string of pia mater continues caudally within the lumbar cistern as the filum terminale internum to become incorporated into the coccygeal ligament. The pia mater within the anterior median sulcus is slightly thickened to form the linea splendens, a connective tissue membrane that provides support for the penetrating branches of the anterior spinal artery. Laterally extending, thread-like extensions of the pia mater (denticulate ligaments) attach to the surrounding dura mater and help to anchor the spinal cord within the meningeal envelope.

9. The spinal cord is perfused by penetrating branches of an anastomotic network (vaso corona) lying on the surface of the pia mater. This network of vessels receives blood by way of the anterior spinal artery located in the anterior median sulcus and the paired posterior spinal arteries located in the region of the posterolateral fissure. At cervical levels, blood reaches the anterior and posterior spinal arteries by way of the vertebral arteries, which give rise to these vessels intracranially, within the posterior fossa. At lower cervical, thoracic, lumbar, and sacral levels, blood is delivered to the anterior and posterior spinal arteries and vaso corona by way of radicular and segmental branches of the posterior intercostals arteries, branches of the aorta. In many individuals the lower segments of the spinal cord receive their blood supply by way of a particularly large segmental artery arising at lower thoracic or upper lumbar levels (artery of Adamkiewicz).

10. The central two-thirds of the spinal cord is perfused by penetrating branches of the anterior spinal artery known as *sulcal arteries*. Sulcal arteries arise with a frequency of approximately 4.6 cm of spinal cord length. In the region of the anterior white commissure, the sulcal branch commonly turns slightly to one side or the other, penetrating the cord in the region of the anterior funiculus. In approximately 13% to 28% of individuals, the artery bifurcates to enter the cord on both sides. The dorsal and dorsolateral regions of the spinal cord, including the dorsal funiculus and dorsal horns, are perfused by penetrating branches of the paired posterior spinal arteries. There are anastomotic connections between the anterior spinal artery and the posterior spinal arteries on the surface of the cord and within the substance of the cord in the region of the dorsal horns in so-called *watershed* areas.

RETICULAR FORMATION

Key Points

1. The term *reticular formation* refers to a phylogenetically old group of neurons extending from the brainstem through the diencephalon that, through their influence on other cell populations, help regulate various bodily functions including the conscious state.

2. The brainstem reticular formation can be divided into three regions based on histological, neurochemical, and functional criteria. Using histological criteria, the three regions are referred to as the *raphe, magnocellular,* and *parvocellular regions.* The raphe region lies bilaterally along the midline of the brainstem and is composed of cells that project axons rostrally and/or caudally. The magnocellular region occupies the medial two-thirds of the brainstem tegmentum. This region is characterized by nuclei containing relatively large cell bodies with relatively long axons. The axons of these cells carry nerve impulses away from the reticular formation (reticular formation efferent cells). The parvocellular region occupies the lateral one-third of the brainstem tegmentum. This region is characterized by areas containing relatively small nerve cell bodies with relatively short axons. The cells in this region receive synaptic input from cells outside the reticular formation (reticular formation afferent cells) (Figure 1-4).

3. The cells of the reticular formation are characterized by axons having large numbers of collateral branches that distribute widely throughout the CNS.

4. The reticular formation as an anatomical entity receives synaptic input by way of collateral branches of all the so-called sensory pathways (general and special) and from cell groups including the hypothalamus and basal nuclei. Synaptic input to the reticular function terminates largely in the small cell nuclei of the lateral one-third of the brainstem.

5. The output cells of the reticular formation are found chiefly in the large cell nuclei of the medial two-thirds of the brainstem. Output from the reticular formation is derived largely from noradrenergic cells in the locus ceruleus, serotonergic cells of the raphe nuclei, and dopaminergic cells of the ventral tegmental nuclei in the midbrain. Axons of these cells project rostrally to nuclei of the diencephalon and telencephalon by way of the medial forebrain bundle and caudally to the brainstem and spinal cord by way of reticulospinal pathways (Figure 1-5).

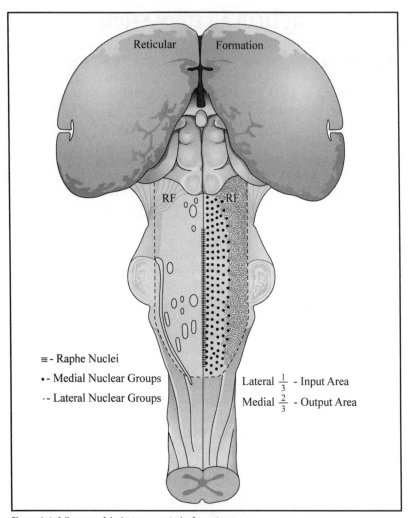

Figure 1-4: Cell groups of the brainstem reticular formation.

6. Lesions involving the reticular formation are frequently associated with death or alterations in consciousness (level of consciousness).

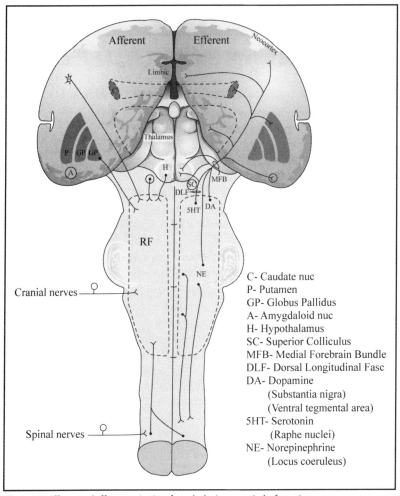

Figure 1-5: Afferent and efferent projections from the brainstem reticular formation.

PERIPHERAL NERVOUS SYSTEM— STRUCTURE AND ORGANIZATION

Key Points

1. The PNS is usually described as consisting of those parts of the nervous system that are outside the brain and spinal cord. Functionally,

this includes the axons of efferent neurons, the peripheral and central processes of afferent cells, and the neural crest-derived postganglionic cells of the autonomic nervous system. Spinal nerves and cranial nerves are considered part of the PNS.

2. Anatomically, the PNS includes the dorsal root and rootlets, the ventral root and rootlets, the dorsal root ganglion, the spinal nerve and all of its branches (ie, dorsal and ventral rami), and the paravertebral and prevertebral ganglia of the autonomic nervous system and their branches (ie, gray and white rami, visceral branches, and splanchnic nerves).

3. Functionally, the PNS consists of nerve cells and their processes, which are involved in transmitting nerve impulses to and from the CNS. Somatic and visceral afferent nerve cells transmit impulses toward the CNS, while somatic and visceral efferent cells transmit impulses away from the CNS.

4. Afferent and efferent fibers vary in diameter and are both myelinated and unmyelinated. Eighty percent of the axons in the PNS are unmyelinated and 80% of these are afferent. Myelin in the PNS is produced by Schwann cells. The term *internodal segment* refers to the length of a single axon between two adjacent nodes of Ranvier. An internodal segment is that length of axon that is myelinated by a single Schwann cell. The larger diameter axons typically have thicker myelin sheaths with longer internodal segments and consequently faster conduction velocities. Axons in the PNS are classified using a system based on conduction velocity. Diseases that affect Schwann cells that result in a breakdown and loss of the myelin sheath are characterized by a decrease in conduction velocity detectable by neurophysiologic testing.

5. Individual peripheral nerve fibers are frequently embedded in a thin matrix of connective tissue (collagen fibers and fibroblasts) referred to as endoneurium. Functionally and anatomically related bundles of axons are enclosed in a water-tight connective tissue membrane referred to as *perineurium*. Fibers enclosed within a perineurial membrane constitute a *fascicle*. The perineurial membrane of peripheral nerves constitutes a *barrier*, inside of which the ionic environment is carefully regulated. Over the length of a peripheral nerve, axons may shift location between neighboring fascicles. Collections of fascicles are enclosed in a thickened connective tissue sheath known as *epineurium*. The epineurial sheath is typically thicker in regions where the nerve crosses a joint over a bony prominence.

6. The blood supply to peripheral nerves is derived from local blood vessels and is referred to as the *vasa nervorum*. Vessels course longitudinally within the nerve both outside and within the perineurial sheath.

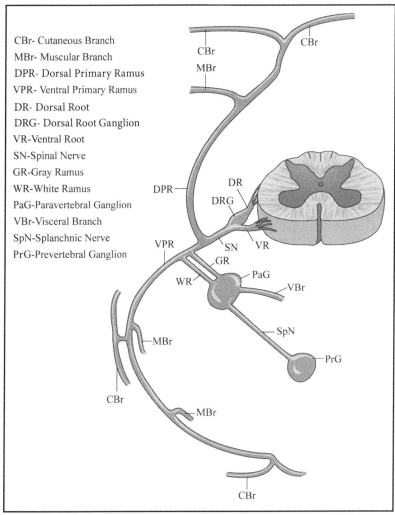

Figure 1-6: Peripheral nervous system structures associated with the spinal cord.

7. The grossly identifiable structures of the PNS include the dorsal and ventral roots and rootlets; dorsal root ganglia; spinal nerves; dorsal and ventral primary rami and their muscular and cutaneous branches; white and gray rami communicans; prevertebral and paravertebral ganglia; visceral branches of autonomic ganglia; and splanchnic nerves (Figure 1-6).

8. A plexus in the PNS is a structure in which afferent and efferent fibers from different spinal segments intermingle. The brachial and lumbosacral plexuses are formed by afferent and efferent fibers that innervate the upper and lower limbs respectively. Autonomic fibers frequently form plexuses that innervate target structures (ie, cardiac plexus, celiac plexus).

9. Spinal nerves of spinal cord segments that contribute to the brachial plexus (C5- T1) and lumbosacral plexus (L2-S2) divide into dorsal and ventral primary rami. The ventral primary rami of these segments then contribute to the formation of the plexuses, serving as the roots of the brachial and lumbosacral plexuses.

10. Cranial nerves (with the exception of the olfactory nerve and the optic nerve) are classified as peripheral nerves. Microscopically, cranial nerves and spinal nerves are the same. Functionally, some of these (CN III-XII) are classified as purely sensory, some as purely motor, and others as mixed (even though all are likely composed of both afferent and efferent cell processes).

PERIPHERAL NERVOUS SYSTEM— AFFERENT CELLS

Key Points

1. Afferent cells transmit nerve impulses toward the CNS and are embryologically derived from the neural crest. Most afferent cells are pseudounipolar in shape with a small number (those associated with the special senses) being bipolar. The parts of an afferent cell are the cell body and two processes: the central process and the peripheral process, both of which demonstrate the histological characteristics of an axon, meaning that both transmit action potentials.

2. The cell bodies of spinal afferent cells are located in dorsal root ganglia. (Cranial afferent cells will be considered in detail in subsequent sections dealing specifically with the cranial nerves.) The peripheral process extends from the cell body forming first, part of the spinal nerve. These fibers then pass into either the dorsal or ventral primary ramus, and subsequently distribute to their target site or structure by way of a terminal (muscular, cutaneous, or visceral) branch. The central process extends from the cell body toward the CNS and forms the dorsal root, which subsequently divides to form several dorsal rootlets. These fibers enter the spinal cord in the region of the dorsal

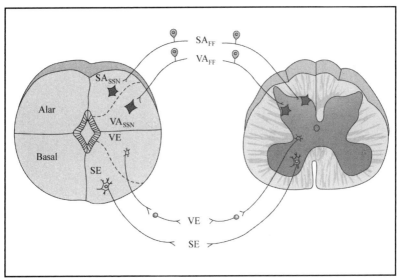

Figure 1-7: Afferent cell types of the spinal cord. SA_{FF}=somatic afferent cell, VA_{FF}=visceral afferent cell.

root entry zone (DREZ) and terminate on specific cell populations, either in the gray matter of the spinal cord or in the nuclei of the dorsal columns located in the caudal part of the medulla oblongata.

3. Embryologically, afferent cells are of two major types: somatic afferent cells and visceral afferent cells. Somatic afferent cells transmit impulses toward the CNS from tissues derived from ectoderm and somatic mesoderm, while visceral afferent cells transmit information from tissues derived from endoderm and splanchnic mesoderm (Figures 1-7 and 1-8).

4. The peripheral processes of somatic afferent cells are found in both muscular and cutaneous branches of both the dorsal and ventral primary rami. Somatic afferent fibers in muscular branches transmit from the connective tissue layers of a muscle, relaying impulses that may give rise to perceptual experiences such as pain and muscle cramps, and from specialized receptors (muscle spindles and golgi tendon organs) located in the muscle innervated. These receptors play a role in the maintenance and regulation of muscle tone and in contractile functions of the muscle. Somatic afferent fibers in cutaneous branches end either as free nerve endings or as encapsulated nerve endings (referring to the fact that they innervate specialized receptors embedded in the dermal layer of the skin). Free nerve endings, sometimes

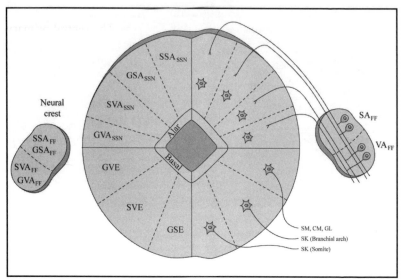

Figure 1-8: Afferent cell types of the brainstem (SA$_{FF}$=somatic afferent cell, VA$_{FF}$=visceral afferent cell).

referred to as *nociceptors*, are classified as high threshold receptors and are associated with conduction velocities in the range of 0.5 to 2.0 m/sec. Impulse transmission along these somatic afferent fibers is associated with the perception of thermal stimuli and the experience of pain. Encapsulated nerve endings, sometimes referred to as *non-nociceptors*, are classified as low threshold receptors and are associated with conduction velocities ranging from 12 to 70 m/sec. Impulse transmission along these somatic afferent fibers is commonly associated with the ability to differentiate among different textures and materials. These receptors and peripheral fibers are also important in providing neural information to brain regions and structures that influence fine motor control.

5. The peripheral processes of visceral afferent cells pass through the spinal nerve and proximal part of the ventral primary ramus before entering the white ramus communicans to reach the paravertebral (sympathetic chain) ganglion. The axons pass through the ganglion (without synapse) to become incorporated into either a visceral branch or a splanchnic nerve. Visceral afferent fibers innervate receptors located predominantly in visceral organs of the thorax, abdomen, and perineum, including the visceral peritoneum and visceral pleura.

6. The brachial plexus and lumbosacral plexus are each formed by the ventral primary rami of specific spinal nerves. The ventral primary rami of C5-T1 contribute (intermingle) to form the brachial plexus and those of L2-S2 contribute (intermingle) to form the lumbosacral plexus. These rami are often referred to as the *roots* or *preplexus roots* of the plexus. Somatic afferent fibers found in a single preplexus root provide sensory innervation to an area of skin referred to as a *radicular dermatome*. Somatic afferent fibers found in a single postplexus nerve innervate an area of skin referred to as a *peripheral nerve dermatome*. Familiarity with the differences between these two sensory innervation patterns facilitates identification and differentiation of peripheral nerve lesions that affect nerve roots (radiculopathies) from those that affect particular peripheral nerves (neuropathies).

7. Conduction velocity along the peripheral process of afferent cells varies widely. Somatic afferent fibers that innervate muscle spindles transmit at two velocities: Type Ia somatic afferent fibers that innervate the primary ending transmit at a rate of 70 to 120 m/sec, and type II fibers that innervate the secondary ending transmit at a rate of 30 to 70 m/sec. Type II somatic afferent fibers that innervate the Golgi tendon organ transmit at a rate of 70 to 120 m/sec. Aβ somatic afferent fibers that innervate low threshold cutaneous receptors transmit at a rate of 30 to 70 m/sec. Aδ somatic afferent fibers that innervate high threshold receptors transmit at a rate of 12 to 30 m/sec. Unmyelinated C fibers that transmit impulses in response to tissue damaging stimuli transmit nerve impulses at a rate of 0.5 to 2 m/sec. Interestingly, most (80%) of the fibers in a typical peripheral nerve are unmyelinated, with 80% of these being afferent nerve fibers (C fibers). Visceral afferent cells transmit at rates generally less than 15 m/sec.

8. Afferent fibers of different diameters are intermixed in peripheral nerves, plexuses, and in the more distal part of the dorsal root. Near the surface of the spinal cord, the more heavily myelinated fibers tend to migrate to a more dorsal position in the dorsal rootlet, while the unmyelinated and thinly myelinated fibers tend to be located in the more ventral portion within the dorsal rootlet. These relationships are preserved as the axons enter the spinal cord.

9. Myelinated afferent nerve fibers (1a, 1b, II, Aβ, Aδ fibers) terminate peripherally by innervating a specialized connective tissue receptor. These nerve endings are thus commonly referred to as *encapsulated nerve endings*. The function of these specialized receptor structures is basically to lower the threshold of depolarization. Encapsulated nerve endings are frequently referred to as *low threshold receptors*.

10. Unmyelinated afferent nerve fibers (C fibers) terminate peripherally as "free nerve endings," (ie, they are typically not associated with specialized receptor cells). The distal-most tip of an unmyelinated afferent fiber is sometimes referred to as an *unencapsulated* nerve ending. Unencapsulated nerve endings are commonly referred to as *high threshold receptors*. These nerve cells are most easily depolarized by changes in the local ionic microenvironment (chemical energy), thermal changes in the local environment (thermal energy), and physical distortion (mechanical energy). They are particularly responsive to any stimulus that produces tissue damage or injury (nociceptive stimuli) and are thus referred to as *nociceptors*.

11. Injuries or disease processes that affect afferent nerve cells or their fibers deprive the CNS of afferent input from those areas of the body innervated by the damaged axons. The effects of such a loss include reduced or altered sensory experience, alterations in certain types of reflex responses, and impairment of muscle tone and motor behavior.

12. Transection of a peripheral nerve (a collection of axons) results in histologically identifiable changes both distal and proximal to the injury site. Distally, there is dissolution and disorganization of the axonal membrane, cytoskeletal elements, and Schwann cell layers. At the peripheral end of the axon, there is separation from the end organ (sensory receptor or muscle fiber) where such end organs exist. The term *Wallerian degeneration* is used to refer to the morphologic changes that occur distal to the site of injury (ie, in those parts of the neuron that are separated from the cell body). Proximally, the axon undergoes similar degenerative changes extending essentially to the closest, uninjured node of Ranvier. Within the nerve cell body, there are three definable changes: 1) swelling of the cell body due to the influx of extracellular fluid; 2) displacement of the nucleus to the periphery of the cell body, away from the axon hillock; and 3) loss of basophilic staining (chromatolysis) suggestive of an increase in metabolic activity associated with the process of cell repair.

PERIPHERAL NERVOUS SYSTEM— EFFERENT CELLS

Key Points

1. Efferent cells are multipolar cells embryologically derived from the basal lamina that transmit nerve impulses away from the CNS. The function of these cells, in the broadest sense, is to provide motor

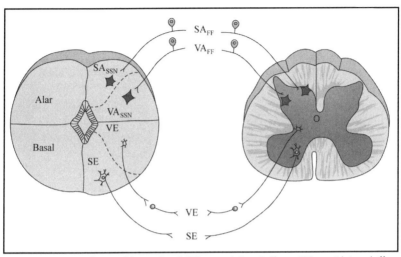

Figure 1-9: Efferent cell types of the spinal cord. GVE=general visceral efferent, SVE=special visceral efferent, GSE=general somatic efferent.

innervation to muscles and glands. More specifically, these cells provide motor innervation to skeletal muscle (both extrafusal and intrafusal), smooth muscle, cardiac muscle, and glands, chiefly exocrine and paracrine glands.

2. Efferent cells are characterized by a cell body and dendrites that lie within the CNS and an axon with multiple terminal endings located outside the CNS. This family of cells includes lower motor neurons and preganglionic autonomic nerve cells. The axons of lower motor neurons contribute to both cranial and spinal nerves.

3. The cell bodies of efferent cells are located in the ventral and lateral horns of the spinal cord and in specific motor and autonomic nuclei in the brainstem.

4. Embryologically, efferent cells are classified according to their relative position with respect to the brainstem ventricles or central canal of the spinal cord. Using this system, three types of efferent cells can be identified: *general somatic efferent* (GSE), *special visceral efferent* (SVE), and *general visceral efferent* (GVE) (Figures 1-9 and 1-10).

5. The most medial group of cells is referred to as GSE cells. GSE cells are of two types (alpha and gamma) based on their conduction velocity and target structure. Alpha motor neurons transmit nerve impulses rapidly (70 to 120 m/sec) and provide motor innervation to extrafusal skeletal muscles of somite origin, the type of muscles that

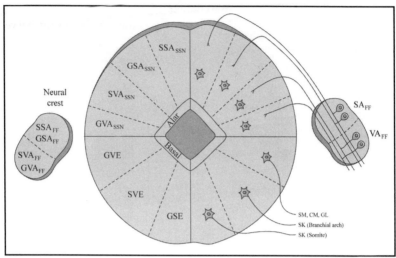

Figure 1-10: Efferent cell types of the brainstem. GVE=general visceral efferent, SVE=special visceral efferent, GSE=general somatic efferent.

are involved in the processes of posture and movement. These cells are commonly referred to as *lower motor neurons*. A motor unit is defined as an alpha motor neuron and all the skeletal muscle cells it innervates. Gamma motor neurons transmit nerve impulses at a slower rate (15 to 30 m/sec) and provide motor innervation to intrafusal muscle cells, the type of muscle cells that form muscle spindles. These cells play an important role in the regulation of muscle tone. Alpha and gamma motor neuron cell bodies are found in the ventral horn at all levels of the spinal cord and in the hypoglossal, abducens, trochlear, and oculomotor nuclei of the brainstem. Alpha and gamma motor neurons synthesize and release acetylcholine, which acts on nicotinic receptors on skeletal muscle cells.

6. The intermediate group of efferent cells is referred to as SVE cells. These cells, like GSE cells, are of two types: alpha and gamma. The target of these cells, however, is skeletal muscle derived from the embryonic branchial arches. Alpha motor neurons that innervate branchial arch-derived skeletal muscles are also classified as lower motor neurons. These cells form the accessory nucleus of the cervical spinal cord, the nucleus ambiguus, the facial nucleus, and the masticator nucleus. The axons of these cells are part of the spinal accessory, vagus, glossopharyngeal, facial, and trigeminal nerves. SVE cells synthesize and release acetylcholine, which acts on nicotinic receptors on skeletal muscle cells.

7. The lateral-most group of efferent cells is referred to as GVE cells. These cells have thinly myelinated axons that transmit nerve impulses at a rate of 3 to 15 m/sec. Unlike GSE and SVE cells, GVE nerve cells terminate on and influence neurons located in autonomic ganglia scattered throughout the head and body. These efferent cells are part of the autonomic nervous system, specifically preganglionic autonomic cells. Preganglionic autonomic cells give rise to thinly myelinated axons that pass out of the CNS to make synaptic contact with postganglionic autonomic nerve cells, which in turn, make contact with smooth muscle cells, cardiac muscle cells, and glands. Preganglionic autonomic nerve cells synthesize and release acetylcholine. (Postganglionic autonomic cells are associated with unmyelinated axons that transmit nerve impulses at a rate of 0.5 to 2 m/sec). Preganglionic autonomic nerve cells form the Edinger-Westphal, superior salivatory, inferior salivatory, and dorsal motor nuclei, all located in the brainstem and the intermediolateral and sacral parasympathetic nuclei, both of which are located in the spinal cord.

8. The axons of efferent cells located in the spinal cord form the ventral root. In the region of the intervertebral foramina, these axons become part of the spinal nerve and more distally, are part of either the dorsal primary or ventral primary ramus.

PERIPHERAL NERVOUS SYSTEM—
RESPONSES TO INJURY

Key Points

1. Lesions or disease processes involving PNS structures can affect sensory, motor, and autonomic functions. Signs and symptoms suggestive of PNS involvement depend on the specific structure involved as well as the nature of the injury or disease. With regard to afferent cells, lesions can involve the cell body or the central or peripheral process. Disease conditions affecting cell processes may involve the process itself (central or peripheral) or the Schwann cell covering (in the case of myelinated afferent fibers). Other disease conditions affect function by disrupting functions associated with the cell body (ie, protein synthesis). Afferent cell impairment is commonly (but not always) characterized by impaired sensory experience and motor function. Lesions or disease conditions involving efferent cells can affect the cell body, the axon or its myelin sheath, or the structure or

function of the synaptic ending. Signs and symptoms are characterized chiefly by weakness and reduced (or absent) muscle tone and
reflex responses. Lesions or disease processes involving components
of the autonomic nervous system affect the function of smooth muscle, cardiac muscle, and glands.

2. The etiology of conditions that affect the PNS includes trauma,
   vascular and infectious disorders, autoimmune reactions, toxic and
   metabolic disorders, neoplasia, hereditary and congenital conditions,
   and degenerative disorders. Some PNS abnormalities are idiopathic in
   origin. Important mechanisms of injury include transection, traction,
   contusion, ischemia, electrical, thermal, irradiation, injection, and
   compression, the latter being the usual mechanism of the so-called
   compartment syndromes.

3. Disease processes that affect cell processes can be selective for afferent,
   efferent, or autonomic fibers, or some combination thereof. Diseases
   may selectively involve myelinated axons or unmyelinated fibers
   and may affect the axon along its entire length or only a small segment of the nerve. As measured in nerve conduction studies, disease
   processes that involve the myelin sheath typically affect nerve conduction
   velocity. Disease processes that involve the axon typically affect the
   amplitude of the transmitted nerve impulse. Disease processes can
   also impair function by affecting cellular functions associated with
   the cell body.

4. Many factors come into play with regard to the question of recovery of
   function following disease or injury to PNS structures. In addition to
   the etiology of the neuropathic process, these factors include:

   • Age and overall health of the patient

   • Location and extent of the injury or disease process

   • Status of the peripheral target organs at the time of reinnervation

   • Integrity of the blood supply to the nerve

   • Other concurrent diseases (eg, diabetes)

   • Delay between injury or disease and repair or treatment

   • Skill of the surgeon when repair is performed

5. Traumatic injuries to peripheral nerves in which axons are severed
   are characterized by several morphologic changes both distal and
   proximal to the injury site. Distal to the transection, axons degenerate
   as do their myelin sheaths, a phenomenon known as *Wallerian degeneration*. Connective tissue elements remain largely intact but may

Table 1-2

Classification of Peripheral Nerve Injuries According to Seddon

Neurapraxia—Conduction failure with preservation of connective tissues structure
    Wallerian degeneration absent
    Large axons more likely to be affected than small axons
    Usual cause—compression or low velocity trauma
    Recovery—spontaneous
Axonotmesis—Axonal disruption with preservation of connective tissue structures
    Wallerian degeneration is present
    Action potentials are not elicitable (nerve conduction studies abnormal)
    EMG shows fibrillation and degeneration potentials
    Recovery—only through axonal regeneration; basement membrane remains intact and aids regeneration
Neurotmesis—Disruption of axons and connective tissue structures
    Wallerian degeneration is present
    EMG and nerve conduction studies abnormal
    Recovery—dependent on a number of factors

retract in both directions, away from the injury site. In the case of the motor axons, neuromuscular junctions with skeletal muscles also degenerate, resulting in paralysis and atrophy of the affected muscles. Proximally, the axons and their myelin degenerate as far as the nearest node of Ranvier. The reactions in the affected cell bodies include loss of basophilic staining, displacement of the nucleus to the periphery of the cell body, and swelling of the cell body. These responses of the cell body are thought to represent changes associated with cellular attempts at repair and recovery following injury to the axon. In some cases, axonal regeneration will be successful and function will be restored. In other cases, for a variety of reasons, anatomical regeneration will not succeed and the nerve cell will ultimately die. Axonal regeneration, under ideal circumstances, progresses at an average rate of about 1 mm/day (Tables 1-2 and 1-3).

Table 1-3	

Classification of Peripheral Nerve Injuries According to Sunderland

TYPE	DEFINITION
I	Conduction failure with preservation of all connective tissue structure
II	Axonal damage with preservation of endoneurium, perineurium, and epineurium
III	Axonal and endoneurial damage with preservation of perineurium and epineurium
IV	Axonal, endoneurial, and perineurial damage with preservation of epineurium
V	Axonal, endoneurial, perineurial, and epineurial damage (nerve transection)

NEUROEMBRYOLOGY

Key Points

1. By the end of the second week of gestation, the developing human embryo consists of two thin cell layers: the epiblast and hypoblast. Near the beginning of the third week of gestation (approximately day 15), specialized epiblast cells begin to migrate from the primitive knot anteriorly toward the prochordal plate, between the primitive epiblast and hypoblast layers, thus forming a three-layered (trilaminar) embryo. These three layers are referred to as *ectoderm, mesoderm,* and *endoderm.* Mesodermal cells along a line between the primitive knot and the prochordal plate (the presumptive notochord) release a neural inducer (NOGGIN) that influences (induces) the immediately overlying ectoderm to form the neural plate (neuroectoderm).

2. At approximately day 18, the neural groove appears as a longitudinal cleft coursing along the dorsal surface of the neural ectoderm (neural plate).

3. At approximately day 21, the neural groove, having deepened since day 18, begins to close dorsally, forming the neural tube. Closure of the neural tube first occurs at a level that will later form part of the cervical spinal cord. Some cells at the lateral edges of the neural groove fail to become incorporated into the neural tube (get pinched off) and remain outside the neural tube as it further develops. These cells form the paired neural crest.

4. The neural tube "zips closed" rostrally and caudally, with closure of the rostral (anterior) neuropore occurring at approximately day 25 and closure of the caudal (posterior) neuropore occurring at approximately day 27 of gestation.

5. The interior of the neural tube is marked by a longitudinally running groove known as the *sulcus limitans*. The sulcus limitans divides the neural tube into a dorsal part referred to as the *alar lamina* and a ventral part known as the *basal lamina*.

6. Functionally, the neural crest will develop to form afferent nerve cells, postganglionic cells of the autonomic nervous system, cells of the adrenal medulla, and a variety of non-neural cells. Basal lamina-derived cells will develop into various populations of efferent cells and alar lamina-derived cells will develop into association cells of the CNS.

7. During development, cell division and migration occur at different rates in different regions of the neural tube. At the rostral end of the neural tube, development is first characterized by the formation of three primary brain vesicles: the *prosencephalon, mesencephalon,* and *rhombencephalon*. These vesicles are formed during the 4th week of development. Later, by the end of the 5th week, the prosencephalon has further developed to form the telencephalon and diencephalon, the mesencephalon has undergone relatively little further development, and the rhombencephalon has developed to form the metencephalon and myelencephalon, the so-called *secondary brain vesicles*.

8. As the brain continues to develop and grow within the confines of the developing skull, several flexures occur in the sagittal plane. The cephalic flexure, a bend directed anteriorly, occurs at the level of the mesencephalon. The cervical flexure, another anteriorly directed bend, occurs at approximately the junction between the caudal end of the brain and the rostral end of the spinal cord. The pontine flexure is a posterior bend that occurs at the level of the developing pons and medulla oblongata. Remnants of the cephalic and pontine flexures can be seen in the adult brain.

9. The human brain is approximately 25% of its adult volume at birth and 75% of its adult volume by 1 year after birth. Growth in brain volume occurs primarily as a result of an increase in cell size (expansion of the dendritic tree and the growth of axon collaterals) and not as a result of an increase in the number of nerve cells.

Functional Organization of the Sensory Systems

Nolan M.
Cram Session in Functional Neuroanatomy:
A Handbook for Students & Clinicians (pp. 41-56)
© 2012 SLACK Incorporated

OVERVIEW OF THE SENSORY SYSTEMS

Key Points

1. The term *sensory system* refers to a functionally organized group of nerve cells that, when activated, results in some type of sensory or experiential phenomenon. While one obvious function of the sensory systems is to provide an individual with a conscious experience of the internal and external environments, an equally important function is to initiate, shape, and adjust motor behavior in response to changes in the internal and external environments.

2. Embryologically, the sensory systems are composed of two types of nerve cells: neural crest-derived afferent cells (cell bodies located outside the central nervous system [CNS]) that transmit nerve impulses toward the spinal cord and brain, and a subset of alar lamina-derived association cells (cells located entirely within the central nervous system) that transmit impulses to target cells located in the cerebral cortex. These latter cortical cells play a role in perceptual experience, stimulus recognition, and the control of motor behavior.

3. The component neural operations of a sensory system are transduction, transmission, perception (including localization), and interpretation.

4. *Transduction* refers to the process whereby energy and forces acting on the body are converted into nerve impulses. The types of energy that can activate a particular sensory system include mechanical, thermal, chemical, and photic. In some cases, energy activates (depolarizes) specialized connective tissue structures (receptors), which in turn initiate nerve impulse transmission toward the CNS. In other cases, energy (stimuli) directly affects the distal part of the peripheral processes of the afferent cell, also resulting in the initiation of nerve impulse transmission toward the CNS. Sensory transducers are commonly characterized according to their threshold (low threshold and high threshold) and adaptation rate (slowly, rapidly, or very rapidly adapting).

5. *Transmission* refers to the process whereby information in the form of nerve impulses (action potentials) is moved from the receptor in the periphery to regions of the brain important in the processes of perception and localization. Transmission occurs centripetally along the peripheral and central processes of afferent cells in the peripheral nervous system (PNS) and by way of the so-called "ascending" or "sensory" pathways in the CNS.

6. In the PNS, impulse transmission occurs at different velocities owing to differences in the diameter of the afferent cell processes and the thickness of the myelin sheath of different types of nerve fibers. Fundamentally, nociceptive information is transmitted relatively slowly, along axons identified and C and Aδ fibers. C fibers are unmyelinated and Aδ fibers are thinly myelinated. Non-nociceptive information is transmitted more rapidly, along axons identified as Aβ and type 1a fibers. Aδ and C fibers are activated by mechanical, thermal, and chemical energy, acting on receptors that are classified as high threshold and slowly adapting. Aβ and 1a fibers are larger in diameter with thicker myelin sheaths and are activated primarily by mechanical energy acting on receptors that are classified as low threshold and rapidly or very rapidly adapting.

7. In the CNS, nerve impulses activated by nociceptive and non-nociceptive stimuli are transmitted by way of two different ascending pathways (Figure 2-1). Nociceptive information is transmitted along axons that form the *anterolateral* system. Non-nociceptive information is transmitted along axons that form the *lemniscal* system. The lemniscal system is formed by cells that comprise fasciculus gracilis and fasciculus cuneatus in the spinal cord and the medial lemniscus in the brainstem. The axons of the anterolateral system give rise to numerous collateral branches in the brainstem and thalamus, thereby providing the anatomical basis for the numerous responses associated with activation of the anterolateral system. The lemniscal system, in contrast, is characterized by the absence of collateral branches between the cells of origin in the dorsal column nuclei and their termination in the thalamus.

8. Axons of the anterolateral system terminate primarily in the brainstem reticular formation and in three nuclei of the dorsal thalamus: *ventral posterolateral* (VPL), *dorsal medial* (DM), and in the *intralaminar nuclear group*. VPL in turn projects to the postcentral gyrus, an area associated with the functions of perception and localization, while DM projects to the frontal, prefrontal, and anterior cingulate cortices, areas associated with judgments about the pleasantness or unpleasantness of a nociceptive stimulus and its relative significance to the individual. Axons of the lemniscal system (medial lemniscus) terminate exclusively in the VPL of the thalamus. Cells in VPL, in turn, project axons to the postcentral gyrus, where non-nociceptive stimuli are perceived and precisely localized.

9. *Perception* refers to the process of experiencing a particular stimulus, while *localization* refers to the ability to identify, with some degree of specificity, the place on the body where the stimulus was applied.

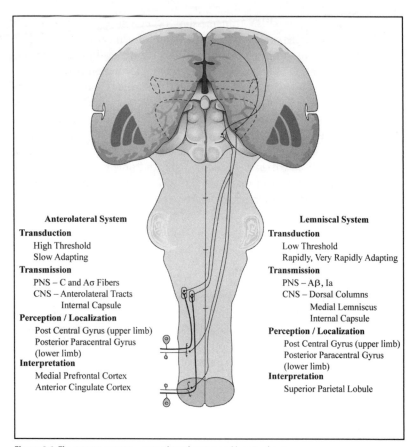

Anterolateral System

Transduction
  High Threshold
  Slow Adapting
Transmission
  PNS – C and Aσ Fibers
  CNS – Anterolateral Tracts
      Internal Capsule
Perception / Localization
  Post Central Gyrus (upper limb)
  Posterior Paracentral Gyrus
  (lower limb)
Interpretation
  Medial Prefrontal Cortex
  Anterior Cingulate Cortex

Lemniscal System

Transduction
  Low Threshold
  Rapidly, Very Rapidly Adapting
Transmission
  PNS – Aβ, Ia
  CNS – Dorsal Columns
      Medial Lemniscus
      Internal Capsule
Perception / Localization
  Post Central Gyrus (upper limb)
  Posterior Paracentral Gyrus
  (lower limb)
Interpretation
  Superior Parietal Lobule

Figure 2-1: The sensory systems—anterolateral system and lemniscal system.

Perception and localization are functions of primary somatosensory cortex, consisting of the postcentral gyrus and the posterior paracentral gyrus. The postcentral gyrus receives projections from VPL subserving the trunk and upper limb and from VPM subserving the face and head. Cells in VPL subserving the lower limb project to the posterior paracentral gyrus located on the medial surface of the parietal lobe. Most of the cells in VPL are activated by axons of the medial lemniscus, suggesting that the primary role of the cells of the primary sensory cortices is to process non-nociceptive information.

10. *Interpretation* refers to the process of assigning specific meaning to tactile stimuli. This function involves the modality-specific, somatosensory association cortex of the superior parietal lobule. The cells of the superior parietal lobule are important in the process of tactile interpretation (ie, the ability, for example, to distinguish a quarter from a dime using the sense of touch only). Lesions selectively affecting the cells of the superior parietal lobule (somatosensory association cortex) or the projections to it from VPL typically result in a deficit referred to as *tactile agnosia*.

11. Projections from the primary sensory cortices and the somatosensory association cortices to the motor cortices of the frontal lobe are important in shaping motor responses to tactile stimuli. For example, these projections help guide finger movements when playing the piano or when trying to insert a key into a lock in the dark. Lesions affecting the lemniscal projections to VPL or projections to the postcentral gyrus from VPL result in specific effects on motor performance typically described as *sensory ataxia*. Lesions involving the somatosensory association cortex that spare the primary sensory cortex typically result in abnormalities referred to as *tactile agnosia*, of which several specific types can be clinically defined.

12. Sensation from the face and head region including the meninges is transmitted toward the CNS chiefly by the trigeminal nerve. Like spinal nerves, this nerve is composed of both nociceptive and non-nociceptive nerve fibers. Nociceptive fibers are relatively slowly transmitting (Aδ and C) and terminate in the spinal nucleus of the trigeminal nerve. This nucleus gives rise to axons that cross the midline and ascend toward ventral posteromedial (VPM) by way of the ventral trigeminothalamic tract (trigeminal lemniscus). Non-nociceptive afferent axons of the trigeminal nerve are relatively rapidly transmitting (Aβ and type 1a) and terminate predominantly in the principal nucleus of the trigeminal nerve. This nucleus gives rise to two ascending pathways: axons that cross the midline to join the contralateral trigeminal lemniscus and axons that remain on the same side and form the dorsal trigeminothalamic tract. Both the ventral and dorsal trigeminothalamic tracts terminate in the VPM nucleus of the thalamus.

13. Peripheral afferent cells can be divided into two major categories: *somatic* and *visceral*. Somatic afferent cells transmit information to the CNS from receptors located in tissues derived from ectoderm and somatic mesoderm. The central processes of these cells terminate predominantly on somatic association cells derived from the alar lamina. Visceral afferent cells transmit information to the CNS from receptors located in tissues derived from endoderm and splanchnic

mesoderm. The central processes of these cells terminate predominantly on visceral association cells derived from the alar lamina. Both somatic and visceral afferent cells are further subdivided into two categories each: general and special.

ANTEROLATERAL SYSTEM

Key Points

1. The main function of the anterolateral system is to detect and initiate protective and reparative responses to tissue injury and to stimuli that if delivered long enough or with enough intensity will cause tissue injury. Anatomically, the system is characterized by *divergence* (ie, the widespread distribution of nerve impulses to multiple regions of the brain, each associated with a particular component of the protective/reparative processes). When activated, the system may initiate any of a variety of responses ranging from simple, automatic (reflex) motor responses, or more complex motor behaviors intended to physically distance the individual from the stimulus. System activation may also result in a variety of autonomic, hormonal, and endocrine responses that are part of protective and reparative mechanisms following tissue (cellular) damage. Collateral projections also reach components of the limbic system, facilitating emotional reactions to the stimuli as well as encoding of some aspect of the experience as a memory. This latter projection is important in shaping responses to subsequent encounters with the same or similar stimuli.

2. Stimulus transduction involves receptors that are classified as high threshold and slowly adapting. Many are responsive to mechanical, chemical, and/or thermal energy. Others respond to changes in the ionic microenvironment that occur in association with tissue damage (ie, cellular disruption).

3. Afferent peripheral nerve fibers associated with the anterolateral system are typically slowly conducting (Aδ and C fibers). C fibers are unmyelinated and typically have no receptor or specialized ending at their peripheral extent. Impulse transmission velocity along C fibers is 0.5 to 2.0 m/sec. Aδ fibers are thinly myelinated and frequently are associated with one of several types of connective tissue receptors (transducers) that serve to lower, somewhat, the threshold to depolarization. Aδ fibers transmit nerve impulses at a velocity of 15 to 30 m/sec. Aδ and C fibers associated with spinal nerves enter the spinal

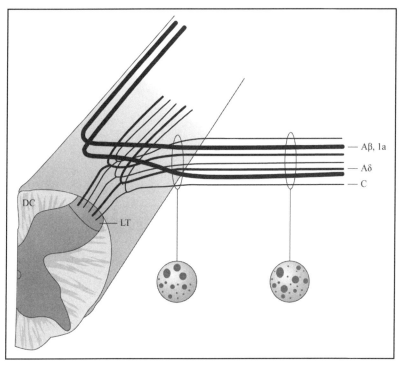

Figure 2-2: Afferent fibers (Aδ and C) of the dorsal root that activate transmission in the anterolateral system.

cord in the region of the dorsal root entry zone lateral to the more heavily myelinated fibers that form the dorsal columns. The central processes of Aδ and C fibers branch immediately deep to the pial surface, giving rise to branches that ascend and descend for a distance of approximately three spinal segments in each direction. These ascending and descending fibers form part of a region of the spinal white matter known as the *dorsolateral fasciculus*, more commonly known as *Lissauer's tract* (Figure 2-2).

4.   Aδ and C fibers terminate in the superficial layers of the dorsal horn. C fibers terminate in laminae I and II of Rexed. Aδ fibers terminate in laminae I, II, and V. The neurons that receive these primary afferent synaptic contacts are mainly interneurons and are the cells of origin of the anterolateral tracts. Anterolateral tract cell bodies are located in all laminae except laminae II, IX, and X. The axons of these cells

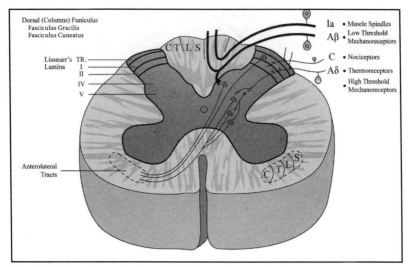

Figure 2-3: Afferent fiber termination and cells of origin of the anterolateral tracts.

cross the midline in the anterior white commissure and collect on the contralateral side, where they constitute the anterolateral tracts (Figure 2-3).

5. The *anterolateral tracts* are so named because of their location in the anterolateral white matter of the spinal cord and because the axons forming these tracts terminate in a variety of nuclei of the brainstem and thalamus. The functional system of which these axonal pathways are a part is consequently known as the *anterolateral system*.

6. The cells of origin of the anterolateral tracts are located in the spinal gray matter in all laminae except laminae II (substantia gelatinosa), IX, and X. Depending on their location and the size of the dendritic tree, anterolateral tract cells receive either direct synaptic contact from Aδ and C fibers or from interneurons acted upon by Aδ and C fibers. Anterolateral tract cell axons cross the midline in the ventral white commissure of the spinal cord, coursing slightly rostrally as they cross.

7. The anterolateral system at the level of the spinal cord is composed of several tracts, the major being the *spinoreticular, spinotectal,* and *spinothalamic* tracts. In the brainstem, these axonal pathways are collectively referred to as the *spinal lemniscus*.

8. The spinoreticular component of the anterolateral system is the largest of the three major components of the system in humans. Spinoreticular fibers terminate in various nuclei of the brainstem reticular formation, which subsequently relay nerve impulses to nuclei located more rostrally and caudally within the forebrain, brainstem, and spinal cord. Ascending reticular formation projections terminate in the ventral posterolateral (VPL), dorsal medial (DM), and intralaminar (IL) nuclei of the thalamus and in the hypothalamus. Other projections may terminate in the amygdaloid nucleus and other components of the limbic system. Spinoreticular projections help mediate autonomic responses to system activation and play a role in effecting responses to noxious stimuli observed in the unconscious patient.

9. The spinotectal component terminates at the level of the midbrain in the nucleus of the superior colliculus. These projections may play a role in activating eye movements in response to tactile stimuli (Figure 2-4).

10. The spinothalamic component of the anterolateral system consists of axons that terminate largely in the VPL, DM, and IL nuclei of the dorsal thalamus. Thalamocortical projections from these nuclei terminate in the primary sensory cortex (postcentral gyrus and posterior paracentral gyrus), frontal association cortex, and striatum, respectively. A small number of spinothalamic axons terminate in the hypothalamus. Each of these projections plays a unique and important role in the complex experiential and behavioral responses associated with anterolateral system activation (Figure 2-5).

11. Thalamocortical projections reach the ipsilateral cerebral cortex by way of the internal capsule. Projections from VPL to the primary sensory cortices are found in the posterior limb of the internal capsule and are important in the ability to perceive and localize nociceptive stimuli. Projections from DM to the frontal association cortices are part of the anterior limb of the internal capsule. Activation of this part of the system is important in judgments about the significance, importance, or relevance of the stimulus.

12. Impulse transmission in the anterolateral tracts can be influenced by higher levels, particularly by nuclei of the brainstem reticular formation. These influences are mediated by way of descending (reticulospinal and reticulobulbar) projections. These descending reticular projection systems may play a role in mediating certain endogenous and chemical-mediated antinociceptive responses.

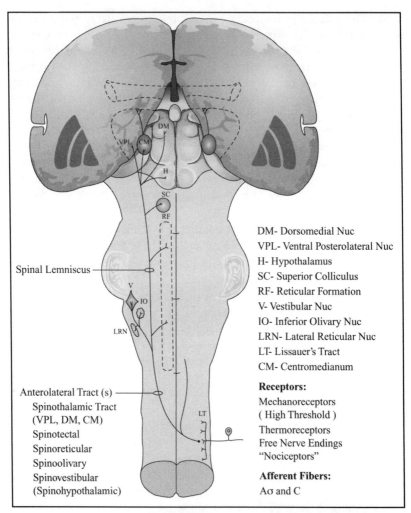

Figure 2-4: Organization of the spinoreticular and spinotectal components of the anterolateral system.

13. Interruption of impulse transmission in the anterolateral tracts results in deficits involving the contralateral side of the body. These deficits are characterized by an increase in the perceptual threshold and tolerance to thermal stimuli, tissue injury, and stimuli that have the potential to cause tissue injury (nociceptive stimuli). On clinical examination, such patients have reduced perception to pin prick and thermal stimuli.

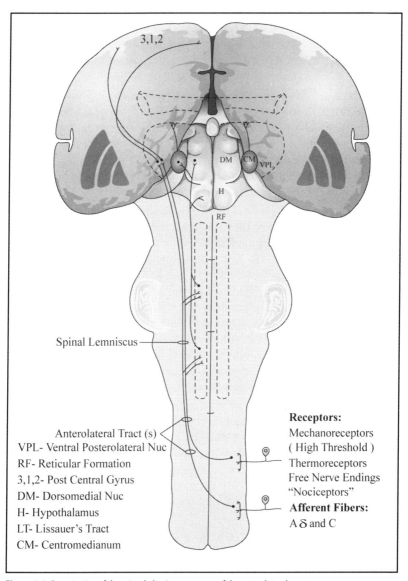

Figure 2-5: Organization of the spinothalamic component of the anterolateral system.

LEMNISCAL SYSTEM

Key Points

1. The main function of the lemniscal system (dorsal column-medial lemniscus pathway) is to transmit tactile and proprioceptive stimuli to the cerebral cortex, specifically to areas containing upper motor neurons involved in the fine control of motor behavior involving both the upper and lower limbs. The system also mediates experience of non-nociceptive tactile stimuli and participates in the processes of tactile recognition and interpretation.

2. Receptors functionally associated with the lemniscal system characteristically have a low threshold and are rapidly or very rapidly adapting. These receptors include primarily mechano-receptors located in the dermis of the skin and periosteum of bone, muscle spindles, and golgi tendon organs. Receptors in skin and bone that activate impulse transmission in the lemniscal system are responsive to low-intensity mechanical stimuli. Muscle spindles (stretch receptors) embedded in striated muscles are responsive to changes in muscle length and rate-of-change in muscle length. Golgi tendon organs (tension receptors) are responsive to tension in a muscle whether resulting from muscle elongation or muscle contraction. Each of these receptor types, when activated, results in impulse transmission in the lemniscal system.

3. Peripheral afferent nerve fibers associated with the lemniscal system are myelinated. Type 1a and 1b fibers transmit nerve impulses rapidly (70 to 120 m/sec), while type II and Aβ fibers conduct impulses at a slower speed (30 to 70 m/sec). The central processes of these fibers enter the spinal cord along the medial extent of the dorsal root entry zone and extend rostrally to the level of the medulla oblongata, forming fasciculus gracilis and fasciculus cuneatus (dorsal columns) (Figure 2-6).

4. The dorsal (posterior) columns (fasciculus cuneatus and fasciculus gracilis) are composed of the axons of pseudounipolar nerve cells located in dorsal root ganglia on the ipsilateral side (Figure 2-7).

5. The dorsal columns are somatotopically organized throughout their extent with axons subserving the lower limbs located medially (in fasciculus gracilis) and those subserving the upper limb located more laterally (in fasciculus cuneatus). The axons of fasciculus gracilis and cuneatus terminate somatotopically in the caudal regions of the medulla oblongata in nucleus gracilis and cuneatus, respectively. Nerve cell bodies that form the nucleus gracilis and cuneatus are

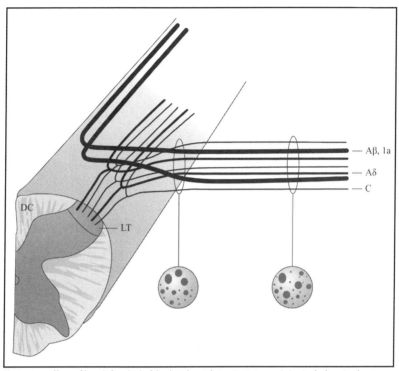

Figure 2-6: Afferent fibers (Aβ and 1a) of the dorsal root that activate transmission in the lemniscal system.

the origin of axons that cross the midline at the level of the caudal medulla oblongata. After crossing, these axons form the medial lemniscus (of the contralateral side). The midline region in the caudal part of the medulla oblongata where the axons of the nucleus gracilis and cuneatus cross the midline is referred to as the *decussation of the medial lemniscus*. Axons arising from the nucleus gracilis cross the midline slightly more caudal to those of the nucleus cuneatus.

6. Axons of the medial lemniscus are somatotopically organized throughout their course through the brainstem and terminate somatotopically in the ventral posterolateral (VPL) nucleus of the thalamus. In the medulla oblongata (rostral part) where the medial lemniscus lies medial to the inferior olivary nucleus, axons subserving upper limb segments are located dorsal to those subserving lower limb segments. In the pons where the medial lemniscus lies dorsal to the pontine nuclei in the ventral part of the pontine tegmentum,

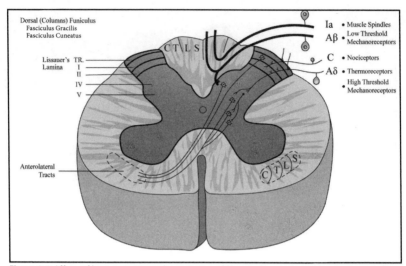

Figure 2-7: Afferent fiber termination and organization of fibers in the spinal part (dorsal columns) of the lemniscal system.

axons subserving upper limb segments are located medial to those subserving lower limb segments. In the midbrain where the medial lemniscus lies dorsal to the substantia nigra in the lateral part of the mesencephalic tegmentum, axons subserving upper limb segments are located ventromedial to those subserving lower limb segments and are intermixed with the thalamic component of the spinal lemniscus. The axons of the medial lemniscus do not give rise to any collateral branches within the brainstem.

7. The medial lemniscus terminates somatotopically within the VPL nucleus of the thalamus. Axons subserving lower limb segments terminate in the lateral part of the nucleus, while those subserving upper limb segments terminate more medially within the nucleus.

8. Axons of nerve cell bodies in VPL lie in the posterior limb of the internal capsule and the corona radiata of the parietal lobe. The synaptic terminals of these thalamocortical fibers are somatotopically distributed in the postcentral gyrus (upper limb and trunk) and posterior paracentral gyrus (lower limb and perineum). These cortical areas are functionally referred to as the *primary sensory cortex* (area 3, 1, 2). Cells of the primary sensory cortex are important in the processes of tactile perception and localization (Figure 2-8).

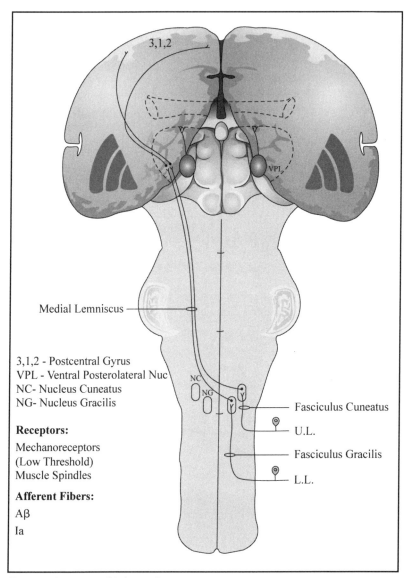

Figure 2-8: Organization of the lemniscal system.

9. Cells of the primary sensory cortices (postcentral gyrus and posterior paracentral gyrus) give rise to axons that project either posteriorly to the superior parietal lobule or anteriorly to the precentral gyrus or the premotor and supplementary motor cortices located anterior

to the precentral sulcus. Corticocortical projections from the primary sensory cortex to parietal association cortices located posterior to the postcentral sulcus are necessary for tactile recognition and more specialized functions, including stereognosia and graphesthesia. Projections from the parietal lobe (postcentral gyrus, posterior paracentral gyrus, and superior parietal lobule) to the frontal lobe (motor cortex and premotor cortex) are important in shaping motor behavior in response to tactile stimuli.

10. Lesions involving the dorsal column–medial lemniscus pathways are suspected in individuals who, on examination, demonstrate impairments in light touch, position sense, vibratory sense, and the ability to precisely localize non-noxious tactile stimuli. These patients also demonstrate characteristic abnormalities in motor performance (sensory ataxia) including a positive finding on the Romberg test.

11. Lesions affecting the parietal association cortices (areas 5 and 7) that spare the primary sensory cortex demonstrate various forms of tactile agnosia. Included among these abnormalities detected on clinical examination are astereognosia, agraphesthesia, and extinction to double simultaneous stimulation.

SECTION III

Functional Organization of the Somatic Motor System

Nolan M.
Cram Session in Functional Neuroanatomy:
A Handbook for Students & Clinicians (pp. 57-90)
© 2012 SLACK Incorporated

OVERVIEW OF THE MOTOR SYSTEM

Key Points

1. The term *motor system* in its broadest sense refers to functionally organized groups of nerve cells that influence the activity of muscles (skeletal, smooth, and cardiac) and glands.

2. Embryologically, the motor system is composed of efferent nerve cells derived from the basal lamina. Functionally, the system also includes cells that influence the activity of efferent cells, namely *afferent* cells (derived from the neural crest) and *association* cells (derived from the alar lamina).

3. According to the so-called *cell column* classification system, efferent cells are composed of three distinct cell types: *general somatic efferent (GSE)* cells, *special visceral efferent (SVE)* cells, and *general visceral efferent (GVE)* cells. GSE cells provide motor innervation to somite-derived skeletal muscles. SVE cells provide motor innervation to branchial arch-derived skeletal muscles. GVE cells provide motor innervation to specialized neural crest-derived motor cells that in turn innervate smooth muscle cells, cardiac muscle cells, and glands. This latter two-neuron motor system is more commonly known as the *autonomic nervous system*.

4. Using a more clinically useful classification system, the motor system is composed of lower motor neurons and the two types of cells that influence lower motor neurons—upper motor neurons and afferent nerve cells. Lower motor neurons and their axons constitute the *final common pathway*. Lesions involving the final common pathway typically result in motor system dysfunction characterized by reduction or loss of muscle tone, muscle stretch reflex responses, and strength. Lesions involving upper motor neurons typically result in increased muscle tone, hyperactive muscle stretch reflex responses, and reduced strength.

5. Lower motor neurons are multipolar cells with the cell body, dendrites, and proximal part of the axon located within the central nervous system (CNS). The axon of a lower motor neuron passes through the pial membrane to reach and form a neuromuscular junction type contact with skeletal muscle fibers. Lower motor neurons synthesize and release acetylcholine as a transmitter.

6. Clinically, the term *lower motor neuron* refers to those efferent cells that provide motor innervation to skeletal muscles that produce movement of joints or skin (extrafusal muscles). Specifically, these

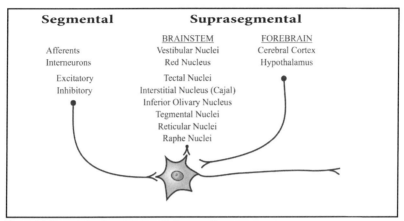

Segmental	Suprasegmental	
	BRAINSTEM	FOREBRAIN
Afferents	Vestibular Nuclei	Cerebral Cortex
Interneurons	Red Nucleus	Hypothalamus
Excitatory	Tectal Nuclei	
Inhibitory	Interstitial Nucleus (Cajal)	
	Inferior Olivary Nucleus	
	Tegmental Nuclei	
	Reticular Nuclei	
	Raphe Nuclei	

Figure 3-1: Segmental and suprasegmental influences of lower motor neurons.

cells are referred to as *alpha motor neurons*, a name that reflects the velocity of nerve impulse transmission along the axon. Alpha motor neurons are distinguished from *gamma motor neurons*, which provide motor innervation to intrafusal skeletal muscles. Intrafusal skeletal muscles form muscle spindles, structures that do not produce movement as a result of contraction. Muscle spindles are important in the maintenance and regulation of muscle tone. Gamma motor neurons transmit nerve impulses at a slower velocity than alpha motor neurons.

7. Lower motor neurons are influenced by afferent cells and a variety of association cells located at the level of the cerebral cortex and brainstem. These influences may be direct or through local interneurons. Generally, inhibitory (hyperpolarizing) effects on lower motor neurons are mediated by way of local interneurons (Figure 3-1).

8. Afferent influences on lower motor neurons are derived from both somatic and visceral afferent sources. *Somatic* sources include muscle receptors (muscle spindles and Golgi tendon organs), cutaneous receptors (nociceptors as well as non-nociceptors), and receptors in other tissues derived from the body wall (ligament, cartilage, periosteum, etc). *Visceral* sources include chemoreceptors and mechanoreceptors embedded in tissues and organs derived from endoderm or splanchnic mesoderm. Only the 1a fiber, which innervates the primary ending of the muscle spindle, makes direct synaptic contact with the lower motor neuron.

9. Cells in the brainstem and cerebral cortex that exert an influence on lower motor neurons are collectively referred to as *upper motor neurons*. Brainstem upper motor neurons are located predominantly in the red nucleus, nucleus of the superior colliculus, the vestibular nuclei, and in certain nuclei of the brainstem reticular formation. These cells influence both alpha and gamma motor neurons. Cortical upper motor neurons are located in the precentral gyrus, anterior paracentral gyrus, and in the prefrontal eye fields. These cells also influence both alpha and gamma motor neurons.

10. Brainstem and cortical upper motor neurons are in turn influenced by three major brain regions: the cerebellum, the basal nuclei, and other areas of the cerebral cortex. The major role of the cerebellum is to regulate **when** in time excitatory and inhibitory influences are delivered to lower motor neuron pools. The major role of the basal nuclei is to help determine **which** populations of upper motor neurons need to be excited or inhibited in order to perform a specific intended movement or sequence of movements. The role of other cortical cells is to help initiate and shape both voluntary and stimulus-driven nonreflex movements (Figure 3-2).

LOWER MOTOR NEURONS

Key Points

1. Lower motor neurons are basal lamina derived cells with axons that exit the CNS and form neuromuscular junctions with striated (extrafusal) muscle cells. In a strict sense, lower motor neurons represent a subpopulation of comparatively large efferent cells with myelinated axons that transmit nerve impulses in the alpha range (80 to 120 m/sec), thus giving rise to the name alpha motor neuron. Alpha motor neurons innervate extrafusal muscles, muscles that attach to bones or skin and produce movements of body parts. (In contrast, gamma motor neurons are efferent cells that innervate intrafusal muscles; muscles that form muscle spindles and participate in the regulation of muscle tone. Gamma motor neurons have axons that transmit nerve impulses in the range of 15 to 30 m/sec. Contraction of intrafusal muscle cells does not produce movement of body parts. Both types of motor neurons synthesize and release acetylcholine at the neuromuscular junction.)

2. Lower motor neurons in the spinal cord are found in the ventral horn (lamina IX of Rexed). Nerve cell bodies located in the more medial

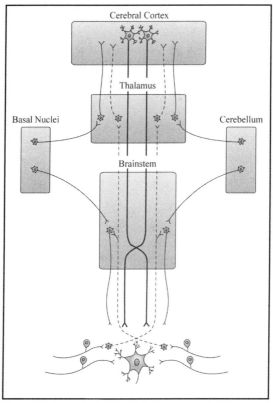

Figure 3-2: Schematic diagram illustrating segmental (afferent) and suprasegmental (brainstem and cerebral cortex) influences on lower motor neurons together with the two major influences (cerebellum and basal nuclei) on those cells.

part of the ventral horn preferentially innervate axial muscles and muscle groups, while those located in the middle and lateral parts of the ventral horn tend to innervate proximal, including girdle, and distal limb muscles, respectively. Additionally, lower motor neurons with cell bodies located in the ventral regions of the ventral horn preferentially innervate extensor muscles, while those located more dorsally in the ventral horn tend to innervate flexor muscles (Figure 3-3). The axons of lower motor neurons form the ventral root of a spinal nerve and distribute to their target muscle by way of the dorsal or ventral primary rami and their branches.

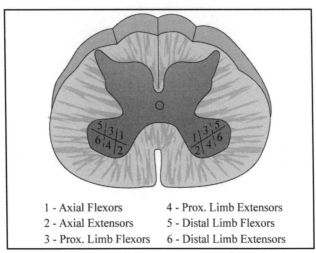

1 - Axial Flexors	4 - Prox. Limb Extensors
2 - Axial Extensors	5 - Distal Limb Flexors
3 - Prox. Limb Flexors	6 - Distal Limb Extensors

Figure 3-3: Schematic diagram of the relative location of functionally distinct population of spinal motor neurons.

3. Lower motor neurons in the brainstem are located in nuclei derived from the embryonic basal lamina. The axons of these cells are found in most (but not all) cranial nerves. Lower motor neurons of the brainstem innervate the extraocular muscles, muscles of mastication, muscles of facial expression, muscles of the larynx and proximal part of the pharynx, and the internal and external muscles of the tongue (Figure 3-4).

4. A single alpha motor neuron, together with the muscle fibers it innervates, constitutes a *motor unit*. Motor units vary in size based on the number of muscle cells innervated. Muscles over which we can exert fine motor control (eg, extraocular muscles, laryngeal muscles, and muscles of facial expression) tend to be made up of small motor units. Motor units associated with muscles not generally involved in fine motor movements (eg, quadriceps femoris) tend to be made up of larger motor units. Relatively large motor units are generally associated with relatively large alpha motor neurons, which in turn are associated with thicker axons and faster conduction velocities. Motor units also vary based on the metabolic characteristics of the muscle cells that make up that muscle. For example, motor units composed of so-called "red" fibers predominate in tonically active muscles, such as those that make up antigravity muscles (soleus and gluteal muscles). Others composed of predominantly "white" fibers are found

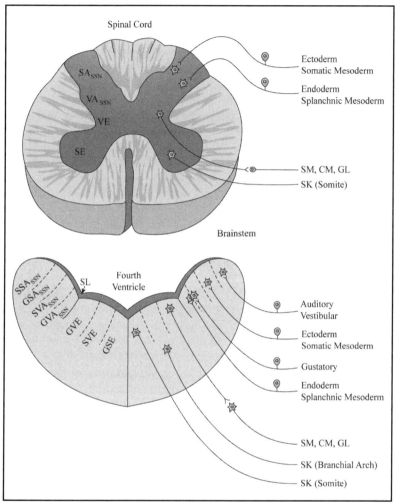

Figure 3-4: Schematic diagram of different types of efferent cells of the spinal cord and brainstem. GVE (general visceral efferent) cells provide motor innervation to smooth muscle (SM), cardiac muscle (CM), and glands (GL). SVE (special visceral efferent) cells provide motor innervation to branchial arch-derived skeletal muscles and GSE (general somatic efferent) cells provide motor innervation to somite-derived skeletal muscles.

predominantly in *phasic* muscles (hamstrings and flexor pollicis longus)—muscles that are recruited when more force or more rapid movements are needed. Finally, motor units differ in their threshold of activation. Lower motor neurons associated with small motor units

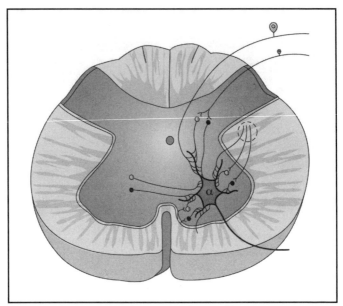

Figure 3-5: Schematic diagram of converging influences of lower motor neurons in the spinal cord.

tend to have a lower threshold of activation and are recruited earlier in a particular movement than lower motor neurons associated with larger motor units.

5. Alpha motor neurons receive synaptic contacts from segmental and suprasegmental sources. The term *segmental sources* (segmental influences) refers to synaptic contacts derived from afferent cells from the same or adjacent neural segments, both ipsilateral and contralateral to the lower motor neuron in question. The term *suprasegmental sources* (suprasegmental influences) refers to synaptic input derived from nerve cells located in the brainstem or cerebral cortex. Interneurons with either excitatory or inhibitory effects may be interposed between the source cell and the alpha motor neuron. Renshaw cells represent a distinct type of inhibitory interneuron in that they make synaptic contact with and inhibit the alpha motor neurons that excite them (Figure 3-5).

6. Gamma motor neurons innervate intrafusal muscles cells, 2 to 12 of which are bundled together to form specialized receptors known as *muscle spindles*. Every skeletal muscle contains hundreds or thousands of muscle spindles. Muscle spindles are specialized

structures attached in parallel with extrafusal muscle cells that are responsive to static muscle length and changes in muscle length. Simply stated, gamma motor neurons play an important role in maintaining the sensitivity and responsivity of the muscle spindle to changes in muscle length.

7. Gamma motor neurons receive synaptic input from the same sources as alpha motor neurons, however, the synaptic influences vary both quantitatively and qualitatively.

8. Functionally, the axons of alpha motor neurons constitute the *final common pathway*, a term introduced by Sherrington to indicate that, in the case of lesions involving these axons in which conduction is impaired, there would be no other way to cause skeletal muscles to contract. Normal function would be affected and the individual would be weak if not paralyzed.

9. Injuries to or diseases involving lower motor neurons or their axons result in paralysis (total loss of muscle activity) or paresis (partial loss of muscle activity) together with atrophy (reduction in size or bulk) of the muscle or muscles involved. (*Note*: The type of atrophy seen with lesions involving lower motor neurons or their axons is referred to as *denervation atrophy*, implying that motor units in the affected muscle or muscles are denervated. Denervation atrophy is typically accompa- nied by specific findings on electrodiagnostic testing. The term *disuse atrophy* refers to a reduction in muscle size due to lack of use, the kind that might be observed in a limb when a cast has been removed after several weeks or months. Disuse atrophy will resolve when normal muscle activity is resumed.)

10. Paralysis associated with absent muscle tone is referred to as *flaccid paralysis*. Flaccid paralysis is seen in association with lower motor neuron injury or disease and may be seen in the early stages fol- lowing lesions that affect upper motor neurons. Paralysis associated with increased muscle tone and hyperactive muscle stretch reflexes is referred to as *spastic paralysis*. Spastic paralysis is commonly seen in association with upper motor neuron lesions.

MUSCLE SPINDLES AND GOLGI TENDON ORGANS

Key Points

1. Muscle spindles are specialized receptor structures located within skeletal muscles that are sensitive to static muscle length and changes in muscle length.

2. A muscle spindle is formed by a small collection of specialized muscle cells referred to as *intrafusal muscle cells*. Intrafusal muscle cells are of two types—nuclear bag and nuclear chain—named in reference to the way their nuclei are organized within the cell. Intrafusal muscle cells are cylindrical-shaped cells with three designated regions: the equatorial region in the central region of the cell where the nuclei are located, the polar regions at each end of the cell where the contractile elements (actin and myosin) are found, and a transitional region between the equatorial and polar region on each side known as the *periequatorial region*. Each muscle spindle is made up of 1 or 2 nuclear bag fibers and 2 to 12 nuclear chain fibers. The distal ends of the muscle spindle are attached to the perimysial sheath of an extrafusal muscle cell. As a result, muscles spindles are attached in parallel with the extrafusal muscle fibers with which they are associated.

3. Muscle spindles are innervated by both efferent and afferent nerve cells. The efferent nerve cells are associated with axons that transmit nerve impulses at 15 to 30 m/sec and are referred to as *gamma motor neurons*. Gamma motor neuron axons form neuromuscular junctions at the polar ends of the intrafusal muscle cell and use acetylcholine as a neurotransmitter. The receptor regions of the muscle spindle are the equatorial and periequatorial regions. Two different afferent nerve endings are found in those regions, the activation of which results in information being transmitted toward the CNS. *Primary* endings are located at the equatorial region of each intrafusal muscle cell and *secondary* endings are located in the periequatorial regions. The primary ending is responsive to change in length and rate of change in length of the muscle spindle. Nerve impulses transmitted toward the CNS when the primary ending is depolarized travel at 70 to 120 m/sec along 1a peripheral nerve fibers. The secondary ending is responsive to changes in length only. Nerve impulses transmitted toward the CNS when the secondary ending is depolarized travel at 30 to 70 m/sec along type II peripheral nerve fibers (Figure 3-6).

4. The central processes of type 1a and II fibers enter the CNS by way of the dorsal root or appropriate cranial nerve. Those associated with spinal nerves give rise to collateral branches within the spinal cord that terminate in several different regions of the spinal cord and brainstem, including local interneurons, lower motor neurons, cells that project to the cerebellum, and cells that form the dorsal column nuclei (nucleus gracilis and cuneatus).

5. The role of the muscle spindle is to monitor extrafusal muscle length and through its connections with cells within the CNS, help maintain an appropriate level of alpha motor neuron activity in the face

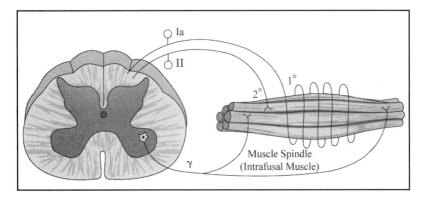

Figure 3-6: Schematic diagram of the afferent and efferent connections of the muscle spindle.

of changing length of the extrafusal muscle. Physiologically, the task of the muscle spindle is to maintain extrafusal muscle length in response to forces that might alter its length.

6. Muscle spindles are the receptors involved in myotatic (stretch) reflexes. The stretch reflex operates to maintain the overall length of a skeletal muscle when forces are applied that would lead to lengthening of the muscle. 1a fibers make direct synaptic connections with alpha motor neurons that innervate the muscle in which the spindle is located. The effect of this monosynaptic connection is excitatory on that alpha motor neuron. 1a fibers also make synaptic contact with interneurons that, in turn, influence other populations of lower motor neurons (Figure 3-7).

7. Golgi tendon organs (GTO) are specialized receptors (transducers) that are sensitive to changes in tension (load) in a muscle. They are depolarized by an increase in tension at the musculotendinous junction, occurring either as a result of muscle contraction or muscle stretching.

8. GTOs are found at the musculo-tendinous junction of extrafusal skeletal muscles where they are interwoven within the connective tissue elements. Thus, the GTO is attached in series with the extrafusal muscle cells that form a particular muscle. When tension increases in the region of the GTO, such as occurs when the muscle contracts or when the muscle is stretched (elongated), the GTO is physically distorted and thereby depolarized. The GTO is more responsive to tension produced by active contraction of the extrafusal muscle than by tension produced as a result of elongation (stretching) of the muscle.

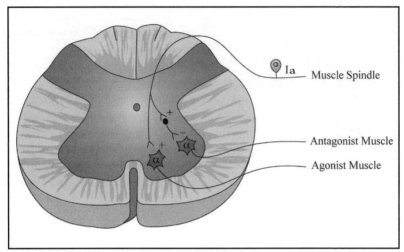

Figure 3-7: Schematic diagram of the muscle stretch reflex arc.

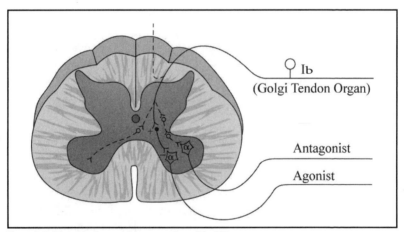

Figure 3-8: Schematic diagram of the connections of the GTO.

9. When the GTO is depolarized, nerve impulses are transmitted toward the CNS at 70 to 120 m/sec along 1b peripheral nerve fibers. The 1b fiber makes synaptic contact with inhibitory interneurons that in turn, act on alpha motor neurons that innervate the muscle in which the GTO is located. The 1b fiber also likely terminates on interneurons that influence lower motor neurons associated with antagonist and synergist muscles (Figure 3-8).

10. The role of the GTO is to monitor tension in the extrafusal muscle in which it is located. The physiological role of the GTO is to counter and balance the effects of the muscle spindle on alpha motor neurons.

11. In neurologically intact individuals, segmental and suprasegmental influences on alpha and gamma neurons are matched. That is, when alpha motor neurons are excited, so are the gamma motor neurons that innervate the muscle spindles in the same muscle. When alpha motor neurons are inhibited, so are the gamma motor neurons that innervate the muscle spindles in that muscle. This neurophysiologic phenomenon is known as *α-γ co-activation* (or α-γ co-inactivation).

MUSCLE TONE

Key Points

1. *Muscle tone* can be defined as the resistance offered by a muscle to passive stretch. Muscle tone reflects the relative (combined) influences of mechanical-elastic characteristics and neural drive to a muscle. The mechanical-elastic characteristics include the weak binding between actin and myosin molecules of skeletal muscle and the binding of the Z line to the M band by the elastic, titin molecule. Neural influences on muscle tone are derived from segmental and suprasegmental neuronal sources. Clinically, muscle tone refers to the level of contraction seen in normally innervated, resting skeletal muscle. The *tone* in a muscle is a reflection of the number of motor units in that muscle that are active at a particular time.

2. Normal muscle tone, therefore, refers to the level of contraction seen in normally innervated, resting skeletal muscle. Muscle tone can be increased above normal (*hypertonia*), indicating the activity of more than the normal number of motor units, or decreased to levels below normal (*hypotonia* or *atonia*), indicating the activity of fewer than normal number of motor units. Both are suggestive of neurologic abnormality.

3. Motor unit activity (and consequently muscle tone) is governed by the balance of excitatory and inhibitory activity impinging on the lower motor neuron. These influences are derived from segmental and suprasegmental sources. Segmental sources include input from afferent nerve cells on both the ipsilateral and contralateral side, as well as small interneurons located in adjacent, functionally related segments. Suprasegmental sources include various brainstem nuclei (brainstem upper motor neurons) and the cerebral cortex (cortical upper motor neurons).

4. Muscle tone (normal muscle tone) is maintained in part by a neuro-physiological mechanism referred to as *α-γ co-activation*. The main purpose of the α-γ co-activation mechanism is to maintain a relatively unchanging (steady) type 1a and type II muscle spindle input to alpha motor neurons during movement when muscle spindles are being stretched or placed on a slack. Simply stated, when α motor neuron firing rate increases resulting in extrafusal muscle contraction (short-ening), γ motor neuron firing rate also increases to cause intrafusal muscle cells to contract and thus take up slack in the equatorial and periequatorial regions of the intrafusal muscle cell. Conversely, when α motor neuron firing rate decreases, resulting in extrafusal muscle relaxation and elongation (lengthening), γ motor neuron firing rate also decreases, resulting in elongation of the intrafusal muscle cell in their polar regions.

5. Lesions that damage the alpha motor neuron or its axon (ie, lesions that interrupt conduction in the final common pathway) result in either a reduction in muscle tone (hypotonia) or a complete loss of muscle tone (atonia). Reduction or loss of tone is frequently accompanied by a similar effect on strength (paresis or paralysis) and stretch reflex response (hyporeflexia or areflexia).

6. Lesions that disrupt suprasegmental influences on lower motor neurons can result in either an increase or decrease in muscle tone depending on the location and temporal profile of the lesion.

7. Suprasegmental lesions that result in a net loss of inhibitory influ-ences on lower motor neurons result in an increase in resting muscle tone (hypertonia). Individuals with significant hypertonia may demonstrate abnormal postures at rest resulting from the strong, sustained, involuntary contraction of a particular muscle, a condition referred to as *dystonia*. (Dystonia affecting the sternocleidomastoid muscle is sometimes referred to as *torticollis*. Writer's cramp is a form of dystonia affecting the muscles of the hand. Dystonia affecting the orbicularis oculi is known as *blepharospasm*.) Other types of supra-segmental lesions result in increased sensitivity of the muscle spindle to stretch. Such conditions are characterized by a more brisk response than normal to muscle elongation. This reflex response is clinically recognized as an increase in resistance to muscle stretch in a resting individual—a condition known as *spasticity*.

8. Spasticity is a disorder of upper motor neurons characterized by a velocity-dependent increase in tonic stretch reflexes (muscle tone) and exaggerated phasic stretch reflexes (tendon reflexes). At least four different mechanisms have been proposed to explain the clinical finding referred to as spasticity.

Table 3-1

Classification of Different Types of Reflex Responses

STIMULUS
 Muscle stretch (myotatic), cutaneous, visceral
 Visual (light), auditory, olfactory, labyrinthine

RESPONSE
 Blink, gag, flexor withdrawal, suck, root

SEGMENTS INVOLVED
 Segmental, multisegmental, suprasegmental

NUMBER OF NEURONS INVOLVED
 Monosynaptic, disynaptic, polysynaptic

REGIONS OF THE NEURAXIS INVOLVED
 Spinal, brainstem

EPONYM
 Achilles, Hoffmann

ABNORMAL (PATHOLOGIC)
 Babinski, glabellar, masseter

DEVELOPMENTAL
 Symmetrical tonic neck reflex (STNR), asymmetrical tonic neck reflex (ATNR), righting, placing, Moro

REFLEXES—MYOTATIC AND CUTANEOUS

Key Points

1. Almost all visceral and much somatic motor behavior occurs automatically in response to various kinds of stimuli. These more or less automatic motor behaviors are often referred to as being reflex in nature. *Reflex behavior* (responses) can be operationally defined as relatively specific and constant responses to a particular stimulus. Reflex responses are modifiable to varying degrees, depending on the complexity of the neural circuits involved. The more simple and direct the circuit, the less variable the nature of the response (Table 3-1).

2. Simple reflex responses, because of their relatively simple neural organization, can be used to evaluate the anatomical and physiological

integrity of those parts of the nervous system that play a role in the reflex response. These parts include the afferent and efferent limbs of the reflex, and to a somewhat lesser extent, the interneurons that may be involved.

3. Reflexes and reflex responses are organized using a variety of classification schemes. While familiarity with these classification schemes is not essential (although it is quite helpful), familiarity with the reflexes themselves is. If one understands reflex mechanisms and the behaviors that are governed by reflex mechanisms, one can more easily recognize clinical abnormalities of reflex function when present and, more importantly, the clinical significance of the abnormal response. Although many different reflex responses are commonly evaluated in the clinical setting, the term *reflexes* generally refers to two specific types of elicitable reflexes: *muscle stretch* (deep tendon) and *cutaneous*.

4. The muscle stretch reflex is neurologically the simplest, consisting in essence of only two neurons: an afferent neuron comprising the afferent limb and efferent (lower motor) neuron comprising the efferent limb. The muscle stretch reflex is referred to as a *monosynaptic* reflex because of the direct synaptic connection between the afferent and efferent limbs of the reflex arc. The muscle stretch reflex is the only monosynaptic reflex known.

5. Muscle stretch responses are elicitable by means of different types of stimuli and are sometimes named accordingly. The two major response types are referred to as *tonic stretch reflexes* and *phasic stretch reflexes*, with tonic stretch reflexes being further subdivided into *static* and *dynamic* responses. The static component generally is characterized by the activity of resting skeletal muscle. The static component of the tonic stretch reflex is evaluated by observing a muscle activity when the muscle is being acted upon by a non-changing, steady (static) force such as gravity. Some forms of dystonia suggest an abnormality of the static component of the tonic stretch reflex. The dynamic component is characterized by the response of skeletal muscle to relatively slow, sustained elongation of skeletal muscle. The dynamic component of the tonic stretch reflex is evaluated by assessing resistance offered by a muscle to slow stretch as might be applied in the routine examination of muscle tone. Spasticity is indicative of an abnormality of the dynamic component of the muscle stretch reflex. The phasic muscle stretch response is elicited by applying a brief, unsustained stretch as might be applied with a percussion hammer. Hyper-reflexia and clonus are signs suggestive of abnormal (exaggerated) phasic stretch reflexes.

Table 3-2

Grading Scale for Muscle Stretch Responses

GRADE	EVALUATION	RESPONSE CHARACTERISTICS
0	Absent	No visible or palpable contraction with reinforcement
1	Normal	Slight muscle contraction with little or no joint movement
2	Normal	Distinct muscle contraction with slight joint movement
3	Normal	Clearly visible muscle contraction with moderate joint movement
4	Abnormal	Strong muscle contraction with one to three beats of clonus. Reflex spread to the contralateral side may be noted
5	Abnormal	Strong muscle contraction with sustained clonus. Reflex spread to the contralateral side may be noted

6. Examination of muscle stretch reflexes is a routine part of the general physical examination. When testing phasic muscle stretch reflex responses, the examiner should pay particular attention to the following reflex response variables: threshold, latency, magnitude (amplitude and spread), and duration. The most common finding suggestive of abnormality is asymmetry between sides of the elicited response. (Thus, skill through practice is necessary to ensure that examiner technique is not a source of variability in the response.) Reflex responses are typically graded on a 4 or 5 point scale (Table 3-2). Lesions in the peripheral nervous system result in reduced or absent muscle stretch reflex responses, while lesions in the CNS generally (but not always) result in exaggerated reflex responses

7. Cutaneous reflexes are elicited by stimuli applied to the skin. Cutaneous afferents effect motor behavior through interneurons interposed between the afferent and efferent limbs of the reflex arc. Thus, cutaneous reflexes are thought to be multisynaptic in nature. The most important cutaneous reflex in clinical neurology is the plantar reflex. The normal response to stimulation of the plantar surface of the foot is toe flexion. An abnormal response consists of extension of the great toe with fanning of the other toes. The term *Babinski response* is used to refer to this abnormal reflex response.

UPPER MOTOR NEURONS

Key Points

1. The term *upper motor neuron* refers to a specific class of alar lamina-derived nerve cells that exert their influence on lower motor neurons. (These cells also, probably by way of collateral branches, influence gamma motor neurons.)

2. Upper motor neurons are located in the brainstem and the cerebral cortex. These cells are the origin of axons that project to and influence lower motor neurons (and gamma) either directly or indirectly though local interneurons. Direct effects are excitatory, while indirect effects can be either excitatory or inhibitory, depending on the neurotransmitter released by the interneuron.

3. Brainstem upper motor neurons are found in several nuclei including the red nucleus, nuclei of the superior colliculus, the vestibular nuclei, and certain nuclei of the reticular formation. These nuclei influence both alpha and gamma lower motor neurons predominantly by way of an interposed interneuron (Figure 3-9).

4. Axons of upper motor neurons located in the red nucleus arise from cells located in the magnocellular part of the nucleus. These axons cross the midline at the level of the mesencephalon as the ventral tegmental decussation. They collect and course caudally through the pontine and medullary reticular formation. A small number of these axons terminate on alpha and gamma motor neurons located in those brainstem nuclei composed of lower motor neurons. Others pass caudally to enter the spinal cord, where they are largely intermixed with axons of the lateral corticospinal tract in the dorsal part of the lateral funiculus. Rubrospinal influences are exerted largely on alpha and gamma motor neurons that innervate proximal flexor muscle groups of the upper limb, with a smaller distribution to cells that innervate proximal flexor muscle groups of the lower limb. Neural influences on the red nucleus are derived primarily from the cerebral cortex (motor and premotor areas) by way of corticorubral projections, the basal nuclei (globus pallidus) by way of pallidorubral projections, and the cerebellum (globosus and emboliform nuclei) by way of cerebellorubral projections.

5. Axons of upper motor neurons located in the nuclei of the superior colliculus arise from cells in the deeper layers of the nucleus and cross the midline as the dorsal tegmental decussation. They collect near the midline, immediately anterior to the medial longitudinal fasciculus

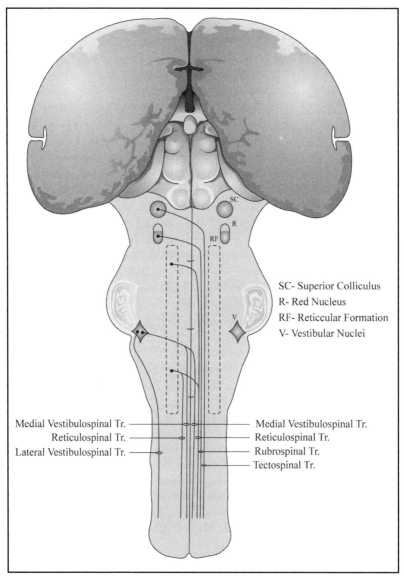

Figure 3-9: Schematic diagram of the origin and course of the main brainstem upper motor neuron pathways.

and course caudally through the pons and medulla oblongata. A small number of these axons terminate in the mesencephalic and pontine gaze centers and on alpha and gamma motor neurons located in the ocular motor nuclei (oculomotor, trochlear, and abducens). Others course caudally to enter the spinal cord, where they are located in the anterior funiculus. Tectospinal influences are exerted largely on alpha and gamma motor neurons that innervate extensor muscles of the neck and shoulder girdle. Tectobulbar influences are exerted largely on the ocular motor nuclei both directly and indirectly through the "gaze centers" of the pons and the rostral midbrain. Influences on the superior colliculus originate largely from the retina by way of retinotectal projections, the cerebral cortex (visual association cortex) by way of corticotectal projections, and the spinal cord by way of the spinotectal tract.

6. Axons of upper motor neurons located in the vestibular nuclei form three distinct pathways. Nerve cells in the lateral vestibular nucleus (Deiter's nucleus) are the origin of axons that lie in the lateral part of the medullary reticular formation and course caudally into the spinal cord, where they lie in the ventrolateral fasciculus of the spinal cord forming the lateral vestibulospinal tract. These axons extend the full length of the spinal cord and largely influence alpha and gamma motor neurons that innervate appendicular (limb) extensor muscle groups. The lateral vestibulospinal spinal tract exerts an excitatory effect on the alpha and gamma motor neurons with which it makes synaptic contact. Nerve cells in the inferior and medial vestibular nuclei are the origin of axons that lie in the medial part of the medullary reticular formation and course into the spinal cord, where they lie in the anterior funiculus, forming the medial vestibulospinal tract. These axons extend the full length of the spinal cord and largely influence alpha and gamma motor neurons that innervate axial (head, neck, and trunk) extensor muscle groups. The medial vestibulospinal spinal tract exerts an excitatory effect on the alpha and gamma motor neurons with which it makes synaptic contact. Nerve cells in the superior and medial vestibular nuclei are the origin of axons that ascend bilaterally in the medial longitudinal fasciculus to influence both the extraocular nuclei (oculomotor, trochlear, and abducens) and brainstem gaze centers, including the para-abducens nucleus located in the paramedian pontine reticular formation (PPRF) and the rostral interstitial nucleus of the medial longitudinal fasciculus (riMLF), and the interstitial nucleus of Cajal (INC), nuclei located in the rostral mesencephalon.

7. Axons of upper motor neurons located in the brainstem reticular formation arise from cells located in small nuclei located in the pons and medulla oblongata. The axons of these cells course caudally through the brainstem and are distributed widely throughout the spinal white matter. Most likely these cells influence spinal interneurons at all levels of the spinal cord. (Other populations of reticulospinal projections exert their influence of preganglionic sympathetic and preganglionic parasympathetic cells of the autonomic nervous system. These cells are usually not classified as brainstem upper motor neurons.)

8. Axons of upper motor neurons located in the cerebral cortex arise from cells located in the posterior part of the frontal lobe and the anterior part of the parietal lobe. Those located in the frontal lobe largely influence motor functions (strength and tone), while those located in the parietal lobe largely influence nerve impulse transmission in the ascending sensory pathways (medial, spinal, and trigeminal lemnisci). Effects on ascending pathways may, in turn, influence motor function.

9. Corticospinal cells number approximately 1 million on each side. Approximately 60% of these cells are located in the posterior part of the frontal lobe (precentral gyrus, anterior paracentral gyrus, premotor cortex, and supplementary motor cortex), with the remaining 40% arising from cells in the anterior part of the parietal lobe (postcentral gyrus, posterior paracentral gyrus, superior parietal lobe). The axons of these cells lie in the posterior limb of the internal capsule. Fibers destined for spinal cord segments that innervate the upper limb are located anteromedial to those terminating at lower limb segments. In the midbrain, these fibers occupy a portion of the middle three-fifths of the cerebral peduncle, where fibers destined for upper limb segments are again located anteromedial to those terminating at lower limb segments. In the pons, these axons form the longitudinal pontine bundles. A somatotopic organization is not evident at the level of the pons. At the level of the medulla oblongata, these fibers form the medullary pyramid. At caudal medullary levels, 85% to 90% of these axons cross the midline in the pyramidal decussation and form the lateral corticospinal tract, a descending pathway located in the dorsal part of the lateral funiculus. Those axons that do not cross the midline lie in the ventral funiculus of the spinal cord as the ventral (anterior) corticospinal tract. (*Note*: Variation in the percentage of fibers that cross in the pyramidal decussation is well known. The decussation pattern described above is representative of 70% of the population.) Axons destined to terminate at cervical and upper

thoracic spinal cord segments decussate in the rostral part of the pyramidal decussation while those terminating at lower thoracic, lumbar, and sacral levels decussate in the caudal part of the pyramidal decussation. The term *cortical upper motor neuron* applies specifically to those cells of the posterior part of the frontal lobe that more or less directly influence lower motor neuron populations (Figure 3-10).

10. The distribution of corticospinal axons is not quantitatively the same to all levels (segments) of the spinal cord. Of the approximately 850,000 axons that constitute the lateral corticospinal tract, 55% terminate at the C5-T1 levels, 25% terminate at the L2-S2 levels, and the remaining 20% terminate at spinal levels not associated with either the brachial or lumbosacral plexus. Synaptic endings of the approximately 150,000 axons that constitute the anterior corticospinal tract are distributed more or less equally to all levels of the spinal cord.

11. Cortical upper motor neurons are located mainly in motor and premotor cortices of the frontal lobe (Brodmann's areas 4 and 6). The axons of these neurons terminate at all levels of the spinal cord on lower motor neurons or on local interneurons that in turn project to lower motor neurons. Corticospinal influences are largely upon alpha motor neurons. Because of their position in the dorsal part of the lateral funiculus, lateral corticospinal tract axons influence predominantly distal limb (hand and foot) muscle function. In contrast, ventral (anterior) corticospinal fibers, because of their position in the anterior funiculus, influence predominantly axial muscle function.

12. Lesions or disease processes that alter the function of cortical upper motor neurons result predominantly in disturbances of strength (paresis or paralysis). Lesions or disease processes that alter the function of brainstem upper motor neurons frequently result in changes in muscle tone and reflexes. Clinical signs of upper motor neuron disease include weakness, spasticity, hyperreflexia, and an abnormal plantar reflex (Babinski sign).

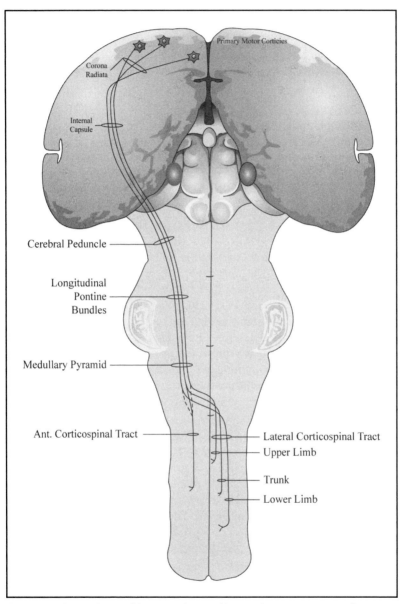

Figure 3-10: Schematic diagram of the origin and course of the cortical upper motor neuron pathway.

CEREBELLUM

Key Points

1. The *cerebellum* is located in the infratentorial compartment of the cranial cavity. Grossly, the cerebellum is composed of three lobes: anterior, posterior, and flocculonodular. The primary fissure located on the superior surface of the cerebellum marks the boundary between the anterior lobe and the posterior lobe. The posterolateral fissure located on the inferior surface of the cerebellum marks the boundary between the posterior lobe and the flocculonodular lobe.

2. Phylogenetically, the cerebellum is composed of three parts. The archicerebellum is represented by the flocculonodular lobe. This part of the cerebellum receives synaptic input primarily from the vestibular nuclei and as a result is sometimes referred to as the *vestibulocerebellum*. The *paleocerebellum* is represented by the vermal and paravermal regions of the anterior and posterior lobes. This part of the cerebellum receives synaptic input from nuclei that relay information primarily from muscle receptors in axial and appendicular muscles and as a result is sometimes referred to as the *spinocerebellum*. The neocerebellum is represented by the hemispheric portions of the anterior and posterior lobes. This part of the cerebellum receives synaptic input from the pontine nuclei (which receive synaptic input from the cerebral cortex) and as a result is sometimes referred to as the *cerebrocerebellum*.

3. Functionally, the cerebellum can be divided into three, slightly overlapping regions. From medial to lateral, these regions are referred to as the *vermal, paravermal,* and *hemispheric* regions. The vermal part of the cerebellum plays a role in motor function involving predominantly axial muscles, whereas the paravermal and hemispheric regions of the cerebellum are associated with motor behavior involving predominantly the limbs.

4. The cerebellar cortex consists of three layers: molecular, Purkinje, and granular. The *molecular* layer is the most superficial layer of the cerebellar cortex. This layer contains predominantly the cell bodies and dendrites of stellate and basket cells, the dendrites of Purkinje cells, parallel fibers (the axons of granule cells), and synaptic endings of climbing fibers. The *Purkinje* layer is the middle and thinnest layer of the cerebellar cortex and contains the cell bodies of Purkinje cells. The *granular* layer is the deepest layer of the cerebellar cortex. This layer contains predominantly the cell bodies of granule and golgi

cells, the axons of Purkinje cells, and synaptic endings of mossy fibers. The cerebellar glomerulus, a synaptic structure consisting of a granule cell dendrite, mossy fiber terminal, and the synaptic ending of golgi cells, is also found in the granular layer.

5. Nerve impulses enter the cerebellum as climbing fibers and mossy fibers. Climbing fibers terminate on the dendrites of Purkinje cells and mossy fibers terminate in synaptic structures known as *glomeruli* located in the granular layer. Both climbing and mossy fibers give rise to collateral branches to appropriate deep nuclei and both are excitatory in their effect.

6. Climbing fibers originate from nerve cell bodies in the contralateral inferior olivary nucleus and terminate by making synaptic connections with cells of the deep nuclei and with the proximal part of the dendrites of Purkinje cells. Climbing fibers enter the cerebellum through the inferior cerebellar peduncle. Climbing fibers are excitatory to the cells on which they synapse (Figure 3-11).

7. Mossy fibers originate from numerous other nuclei of the brainstem and spinal cord. These fibers terminate by making excitatory synaptic connections with cells of the deep nuclei and with dendrites of granule cells (in the granular layer of the cerebellar cortex). Granule cells, in turn, give rise to parallel fibers that synapse on the dendrites of and excite Purkinje cells, stellate cells, and basket cells. Mossy fibers enter the cerebellum by way of all cerebellar peduncles. Mossy fibers in the superior cerebellar peduncle arise from spinal border cells (ventral spinocerebellar tract) and the spinal nucleus of the trigeminal nerve (trigeminocerebellar tract). Mossy fibers in the middle cerebellar peduncle arise from cells of the pontine nuclei (pontocerebellar tract). Mossy fibers in the inferior cerebellar peduncle arise from the lateral cuneate nucleus (cuneocerebellar tract) and nucleus dorsalis (dorsal spinocerebellar tract). Mossy fibers in the juxtarestiform body arise from cells in the vestibular nuclei (vestibulocerebellar tract) and vestibular ganglion. Mossy fibers are excitatory to the cells on which they synapse (Figure 3-12).

8. Purkinje cells are the output cells of the cerebellar cortex. Purkinje cells are excited by the inferior olivary nucleus (climbing fibers) and by granule cells (parallel fibers), and inhibited by stellate cells and basket cells. Axons of Purkinje cells synapse on cells of the cerebellar deep nuclei. Vermal Purkinje cells synapse on cells of the fastigial nucleus. Paravermal Purkinje cells synapse on cells of the globosus and emboliform nuclei, and hemispheric Purkinje cells synapse on cells of the dentate nucleus. Purkinje cells synthesize and release GABA as a neurotransmitter, which acts to inhibit the cells of the deep nuclei (Figure 3-13).

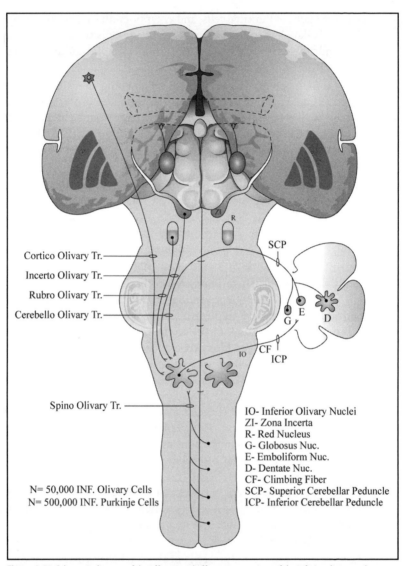

Cortico Olivary Tr.

Incerto Olivary Tr.

Rubro Olivary Tr.

Cerebello Olivary Tr.

SCP

R

ZI

G   E   D

CF

IO   ICP

Spino Olivary Tr.

N= 50,000 INF. Olivary Cells
N= 500,000 INF. Purkinje Cells

IO- Inferior Olivary Nuclei
ZI- Zona Incerta
R- Red Nucleus
G- Globosus Nuc.
E- Emboliform Nuc.
D- Dentate Nuc.
CF- Climbing Fiber
SCP- Superior Cerebellar Peduncle
ICP- Inferior Cerebellar Peduncle

Figure 3-11: Schematic diagram of the afferent and efferent connections of the inferior olivary nucleus.

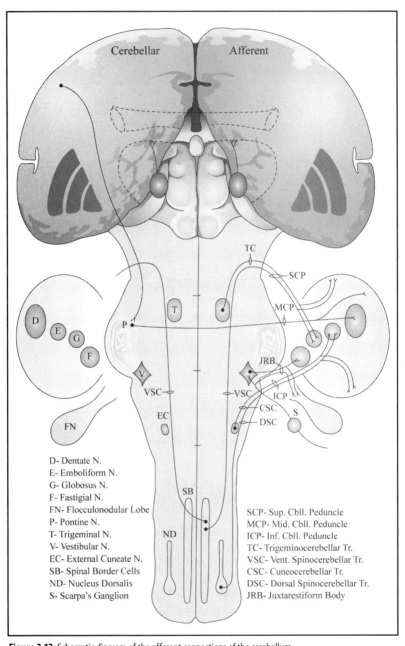

Cerebellar   Afferent

TC
SCP
MCP
JRB
VSC
VSC   ICP
CSC   S
EC   DSC
FN

D- Dentate N.
E- Emboliform N.
G- Globosus N.
F- Fastigial N.
FN- Flocculonodular Lobe
P- Pontine N.
T- Trigeminal N.
V- Vestibular N.
EC- External Cuneate N.
SB- Spinal Border Cells
ND- Nucleus Dorsalis
S- Scarpa's Ganglion

SCP- Sup. Cbll. Peduncle
MCP- Mid. Cbll. Peduncle
ICP- Inf. Cbll. Peduncle
TC- Trigeminocerebellar Tr.
VSC- Vent. Spinocerebellar Tr.
CSC- Cuneocerebellar Tr.
DSC- Dorsal Spinocerebellar Tr.
JRB- Juxtarestiform Body

Figure 3-12: Schematic diagram of the afferent connections of the cerebellum.

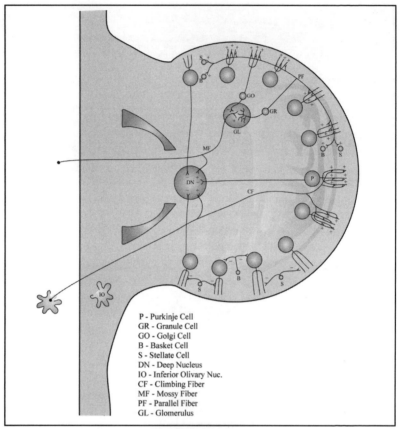

P - Purkinje Cell
GR - Granule Cell
GO - Golgi Cell
B - Basket Cell
S - Stellate Cell
DN - Deep Nucleus
IO - Inferior Olivary Nuc.
CF - Climbing Fiber
MF - Mossy Fiber
PF - Parallel Fiber
GL - Glomerulus

Figure 3-13: Schematic diagram of the intracerebellar connections.

9. Nerve impulses leave the cerebellum by way of axons of cells of the deep cerebellar nuclei. These nuclei are the fastigial, globosus, emboliform, and dentate. Axons of the fastigial nucleus exit the cerebellum primarily by way of the juxtarestiform body and terminate in the vestibular nuclei. Axons of the globosus and emboliform nuclei exit the cerebellum by way of the superior cerebellar peduncle and terminate in the contralateral red nucleus. Axons of the dentate nucleus exit the cerebellum by way of the superior cerebellar peduncle and terminate predominantly in the contralateral ventral lateral (VL) nucleus of the thalamus (which in turn project to the primary motor and premotor cortices). The cerebellar deep nuclei also give rise to projections that terminate in the contralateral inferior olivary nucleus. The cerebellar deep nuclei excite the cells on which they terminate (Figure 3-14).

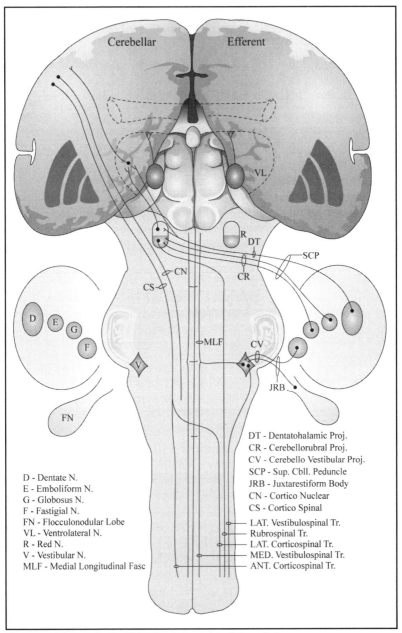

Figure 3-14: Schematic diagram of the efferent connections of the cerebellum.

10. The cerebellum influences motor behavior by way of its effects on cortical upper motor neurons and brainstem (red nucleus and vestibular nuclei) upper motor neurons.

11. The cerebellum regulates the force, amplitude, duration, and velocity of movements by sequencing over **time**, the excitatory and inhibitory influences that impinge on alpha and gamma motor neurons.

12. The cerebellum receives arterial blood supply by way of branches of the vertebral and basilar arteries (posterior circulation). These vessels are the *posterior inferior, anterior inferior,* and *superior cerebellar arteries.*

13. The characteristic feature of cerebellar dysfunction is motor incoordination (ataxia). *Ataxia* suggests the inability to excite and inhibit lower motor neurons (alpha and gamma) in a temporally appropriate manner. The result is muscle activity (contraction and relaxation) that is poorly timed and movements that appear to be not well coordinated (dyssynergic).

BASAL NUCLEI

Key Points

1. The basal nuclei (formally and sometimes still known as the *basal ganglia*) are a group of nuclei located deep within the telencephalon and diencephalon. These nuclei are part of a system of neurons that influence motor behavior through their effects on cortical and brainstem upper motor neurons, and cognitive function through their effects on frontal lobe cortical association cells. Classically, these nuclei include the caudate nucleus, putamen, and globus pallidus. (*Note:* Some authors include the amygdaloid nucleus as on the basal nuclei.) The caudate and putamen are collectively referred to as the *striatum.* The putamen and globus pallidus are collectively referred to as the *lenticular nucleus.* The caudate, putamen, and globus pallidus together are collectively referred to as the *corpus striatum.* The globus pallidus is further subdivided into two parts: a laterally located (external) segment and a medially located (internal) segment.

2. Motor and cognitive functions are influenced by the basal nuclei by way of "feedback loops" involving specific cortical areas and specific thalamic nuclei. Five functionally distinct "loops" have been described, each related to a different type of motor or cognitive behavior. The essential "loop" involves projections from the cerebral cortex→basal nuclei→thalamus→cerebral cortex (Figure 3-15). More specifically, the loop is formed by projections from the cerebral cortex

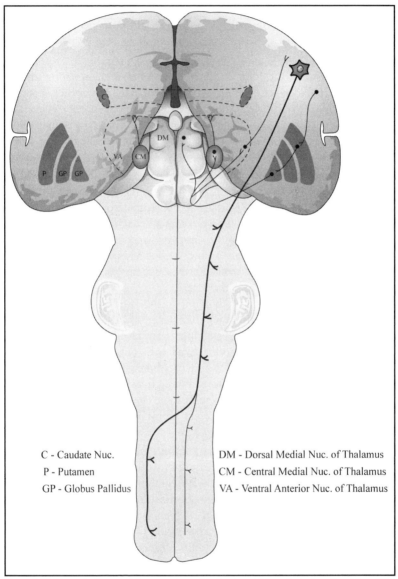

C - Caudate Nuc.

P - Putamen

GP - Globus Pallidus

DM - Dorsal Medial Nuc. of Thalamus

CM - Central Medial Nuc. of Thalamus

VA - Ventral Anterior Nuc. of Thalamus

Figure 3-15: Schematic diagram of the connections of the basal nuclei. Note the basic cortico-strio-pallido-thalamo-cortical "loop".

to the striatum (corticostriate projection), from the striatum to the globus pallidus (strio-pallidal projection), from the globus pallidus to the thalamus (pallido-thalamic projection), and from the thalamus to the cerebral cortex (thalamo-cortical projection).

3. In addition to the connections indicated above, the striatum and the globus pallidus are each reciprocally connected with other functionally important nuclei. The caudate and putamen are reciprocally connected with cells of the substantia nigra and the globus pallidus is reciprocally connected with cells of the subthalamic nucleus. Other less well understood connections have also been described.

4. Two components of the loop system of particular interest are the *direct* and *indirect pathways*. The direct pathway involves strio-pallidal projections that terminate in the internal segment of the globus pallidus (GPi). These strio-pallidal projections utilize GABA co-localized with substance P. Activation of the direct pathway results in increased cortical activity. The indirect pathway is formed by a strio-pallidal projection that terminates in the external segment of the globus pallidus (GPe), a projection from the external segment of the globus pallidus that terminates in the subthalamic nucleus and a subthalmo-pallidal projection that terminates in the internal segment of the globus pallidus. Strio-pallidal projections that terminate in the external segment utilize GABA co-localized with enkephalin. Activation of the indirect pathway results in decreased cortical activity. According to one hypothesis, lesions affecting transmission in the direct pathway may be associated with hypokinesia, while lesions affecting transmission in the indirect pathway may be associated with hyperkinesia (Figure 3-16).

5. The different nuclei that are part of this system utilize a variety of neurotransmitters, the most important of which are acetylcholine (ACh), gamma aminobutyric acid (GABA), glutamate (GLU), and dopamine (DA). The release of these neurotransmitters is carefully regulated in the normal individual. Loss of or damage to neurons that synthesize and release a particular neurotransmitter disrupts the delicate balance within the system and results in the appearance of predictable clinical signs and symptoms. For example, loss of dopaminergic neurons of the substantia nigra results in signs and symptoms associated with Parkinson disease. Infarctions involving the glutamatergic neurons of the subthalamic nucleus result in ballismus. Loss of the GABAergic strio-pallidal cells of the indirect pathway is associated with clinical findings in Huntington disease.

6. *Parkinson disease* is characterized by a tetrad of clinical findings: akinesia, rigidity, resting tremor, and postural instability and is

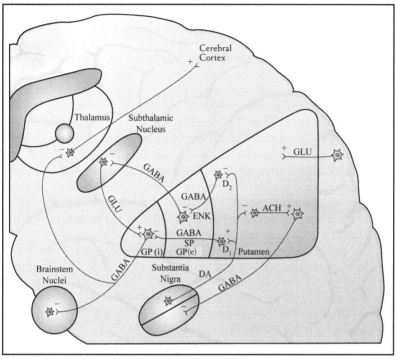

Figure 3-16: Schematic diagram of the "direct" and "indirect" pathways of the basal nuclei including the major neurotransmitters involved and the principal effect on the target cell.

the result of loss of dopaminergic cells in the pars compacta of the substantia nigra. The nigro-striatal projections arising from cells in the pars compacta terminate on the dendrites of medium spiny cells in the putamen and caudate (striatum). Nigro-striatal dopamine exerts two different effects on striatal cells. Nigro-striatal dopamine excites striatal cells of the direct pathway through an action on D1 receptors located on those cells. Nigro-striatal dopamine inhibits striatal cells of the indirect pathway through an action on D2 receptors located on those cells.

7. *Hemiballismus* is characterized by an uncontrollable, flailing type movement, typically of one or more limbs. The condition results from destructive lesions affecting the subthalamic nucleus. This nucleus is part of the indirect pathway. The subthalamic nucleus receives inhibitory, GABAergic input from the external segment of the globus pallidus and gives rise to an excitatory, glutamatergic projection to the internal segment of the globus pallidus.

8. From a mechanistic perspective, movement might be viewed as a means for achieving certain types of goals. For example, particular movements involving the lower limbs (ie, walking) are necessary to achieve the goal of getting from one place to another. Getting from one place to another requires a *motor plan*, in this case walking, which can be thought of as being the product of the development and implementation of several *motor programs* governing the various muscles and muscle groups of the lower limbs. One may view the basal nuclei as important participants in the process of *motor program writing*. The basal nuclei receive extensive input from all areas of the cerebral cortex and, after processing information related to a particular goal, transmit information back to the cerebral cortex, largely the motor cortex, essentially identifying **which** upper motor neurons need to be excited (and which need to be inhibited) in order to achieve the desired goal. Lesions affecting the basal nuclei are characterized by hypokinetic abnormalities suggesting that needed upper motor neuron pools are not being activated, and hyperkinetic abnormalities suggesting that competing or unnecessary motor activity is not being inhibited. Specific motor abnormalities seen in the clinical setting may reflect the delicate balance exerted by the basal nuclei over the motor cortices.

SECTION IV

Functional Organization of the Visceral Motor System

Nolan M.
Cram Session in Functional Neuroanatomy:
A Handbook for Students & Clinicians (pp. 91-102)
© 2012 SLACK Incorporated

AUTONOMIC NERVOUS SYSTEM

Key Points

1. The term *autonomic nervous system* (ANS) refers to an anatomically distinct group of nerve cells that provide motor innervation to smooth muscle, cardiac muscle, and glands. The basic organization of the ANS is that of two nerve cells connected in series. The first cell is located within the central nervous system (CNS). The axon of this cell exits the CNS and makes synaptic contact with the second nerve cell, which in turn innervates the target cell smooth muscle, cardiac muscle, or gland (Figure 4-1).

2. The first cell is a basal lamina-derived multipolar cell, typically referred to as the *preganglionic* (presynaptic) cell. The cell body of the preganglionic cell is located within the CNS. The second cell is a neural crest-derived multipolar cell, commonly referred to as the *postganglionic* (postsynaptic) cell. Cell bodies of the postganglionic cells form ganglia in the peripheral nervous system (PNS). The axon of the preganglionic cell is thinly myelinated and terminates by making synaptic contact with the postganglionic cell. The axon of the postganglionic cell is unmyelinated and terminates by innervating the target muscle or gland cell.

3. Functionally, the ANS consists of two components or divisions: the *sympathetic* and *parasympathetic* divisions. Each division is formed by two nerve cells connected in series, the preganglionic (presynaptic) cell and the postganglionic (postsynaptic) cell.

4. The sympathetic division arises from cells located in thoracic and upper lumbar segments of the spinal cord and is often referred to as forming the thoracolumbar outflow of the ANS. The parasympathetic division arises from cells located in both the brainstem and several sacral segments of the spinal cord and is often referred to as forming the craniosacral outflow of the ANS.

5. Preganglionic sympathetic nerve cell bodies form the intermediolateral nucleus of the spinal cord, located within the T1 through L2 segments of the spinal cord. Macroscopically, the intermediolateral nucleus forms the so-called *lateral horn* of the spinal gray matter. Axons of preganglionic sympathetic nerve cells exit the CNS, pass through the white ramus communicans, and synapse on postganglionic sympathetic nerve cells that form paravertebral ganglia, prevertebral ganglia, or the adrenal medulla.

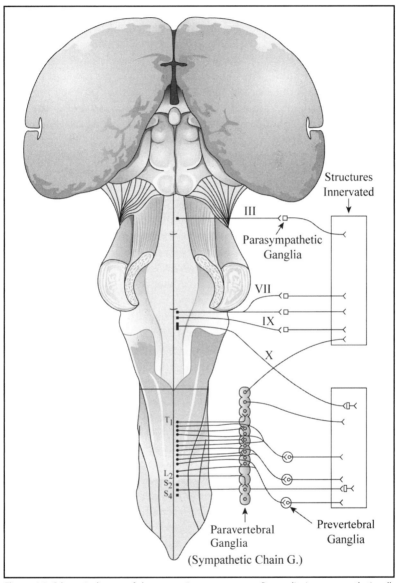

Figure 4-1: Schematic diagram of the autonomic nervous system. Preganglionic parasympathetic cells (closed boxes), preganglionic sympathetic cells (closed circles), postganglionic parasympathetic cells (open boxes), postganglionic sympathetic cells (open circles).

Preganglionic sympathetic nerve cells synthesize and release acetylcholine as a neurotransmitter, acting on nicotinic receptors on ganglion cells. Postganglionic sympathetic cells that form paravertebral ganglia give rise to axons that innervate smooth muscles and glands in the body wall. The axons of these cells course through the gray rami communicans and then either the ventral primary ramus or dorsal primary ramus to reach their target structure in the body wall. Postganglionic sympathetic cells in paravertebral ganglia also innervate cardiac muscle, smooth muscle, and glands associated with visceral structures above the diaphragm by way of *visceral branches* of paravertebral ganglia. Postganglionic sympathetic cells that form prevertebral ganglia innervate smooth muscles and glands associated with visceral structures located below the diaphragm. These ganglia are located primarily in close association with the origin of the major branches of the abdominal aorta. Preganglionic axons reach these ganglia as part of splanchnic nerves. Postganglionic sympathetic axons that arise from cells of prevertebral ganglia reach their target organs by way of the vessels that supply those organs and tissues. Postganglionic sympathetic nerve cells generally synthesize and release norepinephrine as a neurotransmitter, acting on alpha- and beta-adrenergic receptors (Figure 4-2).

6. Preganglionic parasympathetic nerve cell bodies form the Edinger-Westphal, superior salivatory, inferior salivatory, and dorsal motor nuclei of the brainstem and the sacral parasympathetic nucleus located in the lateral part of the intermediate gray of the spinal cord at the S2 through S4 levels. The axons of preganglionic parasympathetic cells located in the brainstem exit the CNS as part of specific cranial nerves and synapse on postganglionic parasympathetic cells that form the ciliary, pterygopalatine, submandibular, and otic ganglia together with a class of ganglia referred to as *terminal ganglia*. The axons of preganglionic parasympathetic cells located in the S2 to S4 segments of the spinal cord exit the spinal cord by way of the ventral root and synapse on postganglionic parasympathetic cells located in or near the organ innervated. Preganglionic parasympathetic cells generally synthesize and release acetylcholine as a neurotransmitter, acting on nicotinic receptors on the ganglion cell.

7. Preganglionic parasympathetic cells of the Edinger-Westphal nucleus give rise to axons that exit the brainstem as part of the oculomotor nerve. These axons synapse on postganglionic parasympathetic cells in the ciliary ganglion, which in turn innervate the pupillary constrictors and ciliary muscles. Cells in the superior salivatory nucleus give rise to axons that exit the brainstem as part of the intermediate portion of the

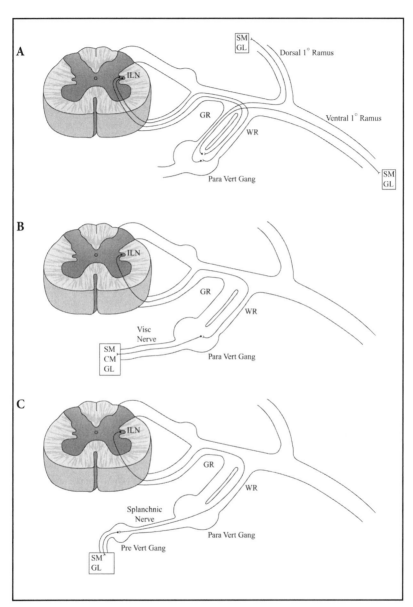

Figure 4-2: Organization of the sympathetic division of the autonomic nervous system. (A) Innervation pattern for target structures located in the body wall, (B) thorax, and (C) abdomen.

facial nerve. These axons synapse on postganglionic parasympathetic cells in the pterygopalatine ganglion, which in turn innervate the lacrimal gland and the glands of the nasal mucosa. Cells in the superior salivatory nucleus also give rise to axons that exit the brainstem as part of the intermediate portion of the facial nerve. However, these axons synapse on postganglionic parasympathetic cells in the submandibular ganglion, which in turn innervate the sublingual and submaxillary salivary glands. Nerve cells in the inferior salivatory nucleus give rise to axons that exit the brainstem as part of the glossopharyngeal nerve. These axons synapse on postganglionic parasympathetic in the otic ganglion, which in turn innervates the parotid gland. Lastly, axons of preganglionic parasympathetic cells that form the dorsal motor nucleus (of X) give rise to axons that exit the brainstem as part of the vagus nerve. These axons synapse on postganglionic parasympathetic cells of the terminal ganglia. Terminal ganglia are associated with the heart and many of the organs below the diaphragm, including the intestine to the level of the splenic flexure. Preganglionic parasympathetic nerve cells that form the sacral parasympathetic nucleus give rise to axons that exit the spinal cord as part of the S2 to S4 spinal nerves. These axons synapse on postganglionic parasympathetic cells that innervate the urinary bladder and distal part of the digestive tract. Postganglionic parasympathetic cells generally synthesize and release acetylcholine as a neurotransmitter, acting on muscarinic receptors in the target organs (Figure 4-3).

8. The two divisions of the ANS operate predominantly to meet different biologic needs. The sympathetic outflow is associated with energy expenditure (eg, when the individual is under stress or when the safety or survival of the individual is at risk). In contrast, the parasympathetic division functions predominantly to drive restorative processes such as eating and digestion, and operates when the individual is relatively at rest. Some target structures such as peripheral vascular smooth muscle are innervated by axons of only one division (in this case the sympathetic division), while others such as the heart and pupil receive both sympathetic and parasympathetic innervation.

9. The ANS plays an important role in maintaining biologic homeostasis. The major neural influences on the ANS are the hypothalamus and the limbic system.

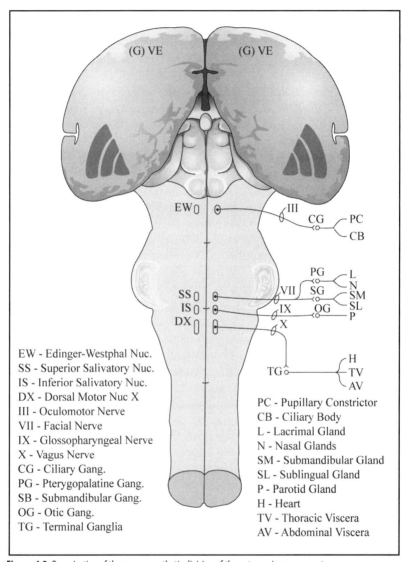

Figure 4-3: Organization of the parasympathetic division of the autonomic nervous system.

HYPOTHALAMUS

Key Points

1. The *hypothalamus* is a small region of the forebrain embryologically derived from the diencephalon (as are the nuclei and fiber structures associated with the dorsal thalamus, ventral thalamus, epithalamus, and metathalamus).

2. The hypothalamus consists of several cell groups (nuclei) located in a small area bounded anteriorly by the lamina terminalis; ventrally by the optic chiasm, median eminence, and mamillary bodies; posteriorly by a line extending from the posterior margin of the mamillary body to the posterior commissure; and superiorly by the hypothalamic sulcus, a shallow groove-like depression on the lateral wall of the third ventricle extending from the posterior commissure to the anterior commissure. The hypothalamus is only several millimeters in width, lying between the internal capsule and ventral pallidum laterally and the ependymal lining of the third ventricle medially.

3. For descriptive purposes, the hypothalamus is commonly divided into medial and lateral regions, with the medial region being further divided into a thin, periventricular region and a slightly thicker paraventricular region. The medial region is further divided into three anterior-posterior regions: chiasmatic, tuberal, and mamillary (Figure 4-4).

4. The columns of the fornix, a myelinated fiber bundle extending from the hippocampal formation in the temporal lobe to the mamillary body, is used to divide the hypothalamus into medial and lateral regions. The medial region is composed of a thin periventricular region located immediately adjacent (deep) to the ependymal lining of the third ventricle and a slightly thicker, cell-rich paraventricular region located between the periventricular region and the column of the fornix. Most of the well-known nuclei of the hypothalamus are located within the paraventricular region. Nuclei included in the chiasmatic region include the anterior, preoptic, supraoptic, paraventricular, and suprachiasmatic. Nuclei included in the tuberal region include the dorsomedial, ventromedial, and arcuate. Nuclei included in the mamillary region include the mamillary and posterior. The lateral region of the hypothalamus, located lateral to the fornix, is also a rather thin area. The medial forebrain bundle (MFB), an unmyelinated, bidirectional pathway connecting the hypothalamus with cortical and nuclear structures of the basal forebrain rostrally and specific

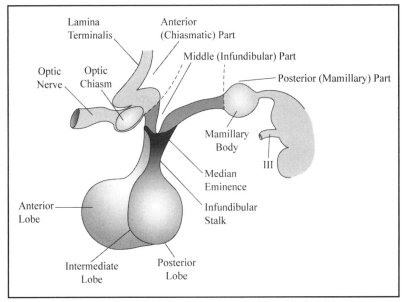

Figure 4-4: Schematic diagram indicating the three anatomical regions of the hypothalamus—anterior (chiasmatic), middle (infundibular), and posterior (mamillary).

nuclei of the brainstem caudally, is located in and passes though the lateral hypothalamic area (Figure 4-5).

5. The hypothalamus exerts an influence on visceral and somatic motor behavior and a variety of hormonal responses by way of connections primarily with the 1) pituitary gland, 2) limbic system and septal area, 3) autonomic cells groups of the brainstem and spinal cord, and 4) dorsal thalamus.

6. Hypothalamic connections with the pituitary gland are directed to both the posterior lobe (pars nervosa) and the anterior lobe (pars distalis). Regarding the posterior lobe, large cells in the supraoptic and paraventricular nuclei (magnocellular nuclei) give rise to axons that pass through the infundibulum to terminate in the posterior lobe where their synaptic endings lie in close relation with the fenestrated capillaries located in this part of the gland. These large cells synthesize oxytocin and antidiuretic hormone (ADH), products that are transported intra-axonally (as Herring bodies) to the posterior lobe, where they are exocytosed and taken up into the nearby capillaries. Oxytocin and ADH are carried by the pituitary veins into the cavernous ·

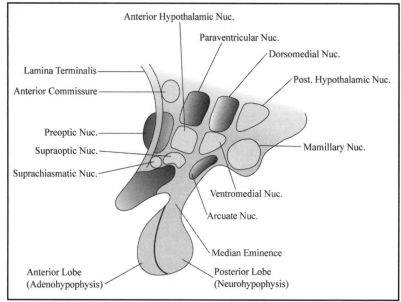

Figure 4-5: Schematic diagram of the major nuclear groups of the hypothalamus.

sinus and subsequently delivered by way of the bloodstream to their target organs. Actions of ADH include increased water resorption by the kidney and increases in systemic blood pressure. Actions of oxytocin include stimulation of uterine smooth muscle contraction during parturition and stimulation of milk ejection from the mammary gland. Regarding the anterior lobe, small cells in the chiasmatic, tuberal, and mamillary regions give rise to axons that terminate in the region of the median eminence in close association with fenestrated capillaries (primary portal plexus) located in this part of the hypothalamus. These small hypothalamic cells synthesize peptides (releasing hormones), which are exocytosed in the region of the median eminence, taken up into the primary portal plexus, and carried into the anterior lobe by way of the long hypophyseal portal veins. In the anterior lobe, releasing hormones leave the vascular channel, passing from the secondary portal plexus into the anterior lobe, where they promote the production of a variety of pituitary hormones. Releasing hormones acting on acidophils promote the production of growth hormone (GH) and prolactin. Releasing hormones acting on basophils promote the production of thyroid-stimulating hormones (TSH), follicle-stimulating hormone (FSH), luteinizing hormone (LH), and adreno-corticotropic hormone (ACTH). Anterior pituitary hormones are taken up into the secondary portal plexus, carried to the cavernous sinus, and subsequently delivered to their target organs by way of the blood stream.

7. Hypothalamic connections with the limbic system are bidirectional, although they largely consist of projections from limbic structures (hippocampal formation and amygdala) and the septal nuclei. The major connection with the hippocampal formation is the fornix. The fornix arises from cells in the subiculum and hippocampus and terminates predominantly in the mamillary nucleus. (Collateral branches terminate in the anterior nucleus of the thalamus and septal nuclei.) The major connections with the amygdaloid nucleus are by way of the stria terminalis and the ventral amygdalo-fugal pathway. They arise from the corticomedial nucleus of the amygdala and terminate predominantly in the ventromedial nucleus of the hypothalamus. (Collateral branches terminate in the septal nuclei.) The major connections with the septal nuclei are found in the anterior part of the medial forebrain bundle (MFB).

8. Hypothalamic connections with autonomic nuclei of the brainstem and spinal cord pass caudally in the dorsal longitudinal fasciculus (dlf), an unmyelinated pathway located in the lateral hypothalamic area. At more caudal levels, the pathway is found in the ventral region of the periaqueductal gray, dorsal regions of the pontine and medullary reticular formation, and near the central gray of the spinal cord. Descending projections in the dlf arise from nuclei located in all three regions of the hypothalamus. Hypothalamic projections also terminate in various nuclei of the brainstem formation. These latter projections are likely part of the mamillo-tegmental tract and may influence nonautonomic functions such as breathing and consciousness.

9. Hypothalamic connections with the dorsal thalamus project to two main targets: the dorsal medial nucleus and the anterior nucleus. Projections to the dorsal medial nucleus are direct. Projections to the anterior nucleus form the *mamillo-thalamic tract*, a large bundle of fibers located in the internal medullary lamina of the thalamus. This latter pathway is part of an important limbic pathway, the Papez circuit.

10. Afferent input to the hypothalamus is delivered by both vascular channels and neural projections. Hypothalamic cells, particularly in the median eminence where the capillaries are fenestrated (where the blood-brain-barrier is absent), respond to changes in circulating levels of various substances. Neural input to the hypothalamus is derived from a large variety of sources, including the olfactory and

optic nerves, visceral and somatic association cells of the spinal cord and brainstem (nucleus solitarius), monoamine synthesizing nuclei of the brainstem (locus ceruleus, raphe nuclei), cells of the limbic system (amygdaloid and mamillary nuclei), frontal lobe cortices and the septal nuclei, and certain nuclei of the dorsal thalamus (medial dorsal). Specialized hypothalamic cells, with cell processes reaching the ependymal lining of the third ventricle, monitor changes in composition and concentration of substances in the CSF.

11. The hypothalamus receives its blood supply by way of branches derived largely from the circle of Willis. Venous drainage is by way of an extensive network of veins that drain into the cavernous sinus.

12. The hypothalamus plays an important role in the regulation of a wide variety of endocrine, autonomic, and emotional behaviors.

SECTION V

Functional Organization of the Cranial Nerves

Nolan M.
*Cram Session in Functional Neuroanatomy:
A Handbook for Students & Clinicians* (pp. 103-170)
© 2012 SLACK Incorporated

OVERVIEW OF THE CRANIAL NERVES

Key Points

1. The *cranial nerves* are peripheral nerves anatomically associated with the forebrain and brainstem. Like spinal nerves, cranial nerves are composed of afferent and efferent axons. However, unlike spinal nerves, which contain both afferent and efferent axons, some cranial nerves consist of only efferent axons, some consist of only afferent axons, and some contain both types of axons.

2. Cranial nerves III to XII are considered typical cranial nerves in that their efferent axons arise from cells derived from the basal lamina and their afferent axons (or more precisely the peripheral processes of the afferent cells) arise from neural crest-derived cells located in specific sensory ganglia found along the course of the nerve.

3. Cranial nerve I, the olfactory nerve, if defined at all, would be considered to be the olfactory fila, axonal-like cell processes of the olfactory receptor cells located in the olfactory epithelium. These cell processes pass upward through the cribriform plate of the ethmoid bone to terminate on cells of the olfactory bulb, a structure derived from the embryonic telencephalon.

4. Cranial nerve II, the optic nerve, is in fact not a peripheral nerve structure, but rather one segment of the axon of the ganglion cell of the retina, a structure derived from the embryonic diencephalon. Specifically, the term *optic nerve* refers to that portion of the ganglion cell axon that extends from the cell body in the retina to the optic chiasm. Thus, the optic nerve is in reality part of the axon of a cell derived from the alar lamina (not the neural crest).

5. Cranial nerve III, the oculomotor nerve, is a motor nerve that consists of efferent fibers that provide motor innervation to the extraocular muscles and levator palpebrae superioris. It also includes autonomic fibers (parasympathetic) that provide motor innervation to the pupillary constrictor and ciliary muscles.

6. Cranial nerve IV, the trochlear nerve, is a motor nerve that consists of efferent fibers that provide motor innervation to the superior oblique muscle. It is the only cranial nerve that emerges from the dorsal surface of the brainstem.

7. Cranial nerve V, the trigeminal nerve, is a mixed nerve that consists of both efferent and afferent fibers. The efferent fibers provide motor innervation to skeletal muscles derived from the first branchial arch, most importantly the muscles of mastication and the tensor tympani.

The afferent fibers transmit impulse to the brain from receptors located in the skin of the face and scalp, the anterior parts of the nasal and oral cavities including the teeth, the cornea, and the meninges of primarily the supratentorial compartment. The trigeminal nerve is sometimes referred to as the "great sensory nerve of the face."

8. Cranial nerve VI, the abducens nerve, is a motor nerve that provides motor innervation to the lateral rectus muscle of the eye.

9. Cranial nerve VII, the facial nerve, is a mixed nerve composed of both afferent and efferent fibers. The facial nerve provides special sensory innervation to the taste buds on the anterior two-thirds of the tongue. The efferent (motor) fibers of the facial nerve provide autonomic (parasympathetic) innervation to the lacrimal gland and to the sublingual and submandibular salivary glands and motor innervation to the muscles of facial expression and the stapedius.

10. Cranial nerve VIII, the vestibulocochlear nerve, is composed of the cochlear division (nerve) and the vestibular division (nerve). The cochlear nerve is predominantly afferent in function and is part of the auditory system. The cochlear nerve provides afferent innervation of the Organ of Corti. The vestibular nerve is also composed of afferent fibers. These fibers innervate the receptor cells of the semicircular canals and the otolithic organs of the utricle and saccule. The vestibular nerve provides the brain with information regarding head position in space and head movements in various planes and around various axes. The vestibular nerve and vestibular system are important in control of eye position in the orbit and head position on the neck.

11. Cranial nerve IX, the glossopharyngeal nerve, is a mixed nerve. Efferent fibers of the nerve provide motor innervation to the stylopharyngeus muscle and autonomic (parasympathetic) innervation to the parotid gland. The afferent fibers innervate the posterior regions of the oropharynx and serve as the afferent limb of the pharyngeal (gag) reflex. Afferent fibers also innervate the baroreceptors of the carotid sinus.

12. Cranial nerve X, the vagus nerve, is a mixed nerve. Efferent fibers of the nerve provide motor innervation to the muscles of the larynx and pharynx and autonomic (parasympathetic) innervation to the heart and the smooth muscles and glands of the digestive tract from the upper esophagus to approximately the level of the splenic flexure of the large colon. The afferent fibers innervate the mucosal lining of the digestive tract from the esophagus to the splenic flexure as well as the visceral layers of the pleura and pericardium. Afferent fibers also innervate the chemoreceptors of the carotid body.

13. Cranial nerve XI, the accessory (spinal accessory) nerve, is a motor nerve. This nerve, unlike other cranial nerves, arises from cells located in upper cervical segments of the spinal cord. The axons of these cells ascend within the spinal subarachnoid space to enter the skull by way of the foramen magnum, only to exit the skull again by way of the jugular foramen. The accessory nerve provides motor innervation to the trapezius and sternocleidomastoid muscles.

14. Cranial nerve XII, the hypoglossal nerve, is a motor nerve. The hypoglossal nerve provides motor innervation to the intrinsic and extrinsic muscles of the tongue.

OLFACTORY SYSTEM

Key Points

1. The *olfactory system* is a phylogenetically old system. Macronosmic animals use the sense of smell to identify food (what is good to eat and what is not), friends and enemies, and partners for mating. Olfactory activation in these animals elicits a variety of automatic (reflex) responses, including sniffing, licking, chewing, biting, salivation, gastric motility, and sneezing as well as more complex behaviors associated with fight and flight, sexual arousal, and reproduction. The system works to preserve the animal's integrity when not being challenged. In micronosmic animals, such as humans, olfactory stimuli elicit many of these responses but often to a lesser degree. Moreover, in humans, olfactory-elicited behaviors are less automatic and more likely to be under the control of the cerebral cortex.

2. The olfactory system is composed of specialized nerve cells (receptor cells) that respond to a variety of odorants inhaled through the nose. Activation of these cells gives rise to impulse transmission along fiber pathways that terminate in regions of the brain involved in the conscious perception and recognition of odors; the activation of autonomic, endocrine, hormonal, and somatic motor responses; and the processes of learning and remembering.

3. *Olfactory receptor cells* are found in the olfactory epithelium located in the roof of the nasal cavity. The epithelial layer is formed by olfactory receptor cells, supporting cells, basal cells, and glandular cells (Bowman's glands). Odorants entering the nasal cavity are dissolved in the secretions from Bowman's glands, thereby facilitating binding with olfactory receptor cells. Olfactory receptor cells are bipolar cells with a cell body located in the olfactory epithelium, a small diameter

axon directed toward the olfactory bulb and a single apical dendrite directed downward, into the roof of the nasal cavity. At the distal end of the apical dendrite is a ciliated swelling, the olfactory vesicle, located in the roof of the nasal cavity. Chemoreceptors are embedded in cilia associated with olfactory vesicles. The thin, central process (axon) of an olfactory nerve cell passes upward through the cribriform plate of the ethmoid bone (as the olfactory nerve) and terminates in the olfactory bulb in a structure referred to as a *glomerulus.* Olfactory nerve fibers pass through the cribriform plate in bundles of approximately 20 to 100 fibers, referred to as *olfactory fila.*

4. Humans are reported to have approximately 12 to 100 million olfactory receptor cells. (Dogs have approximately 4 billion and bloodhounds are said to have a sense of smell that is 300 million times more sensitive than man.) Olfactory receptor cells have a calculated life cycle of approximately 35 days (exact data from humans are not available), after which they degenerate and are replaced by new receptor cells derived from basal cells. (Olfactory cells are one of the few nerve cell types capable of regeneration.)

5. The olfactory nerves (axons of olfactory receptor cells) terminate in the olfactory bulb—the dilated, distal region of the olfactory tract. The olfactory bulb is formed principally by mitral cells, granule cells, tufted cells, and periglomerular cells. Olfactory nerve fibers terminate on apical dendrites of mitral and tufted cells and cellular processes of periglomerular cells in synaptic structures referred to as *glomeruli.* Periglomerular and granule cells are thought to be inhibitory in their effect on mitral cells. According to estimates in humans, each olfactory bulb contains approximately 12,000 glomeruli. These structures receive convergent input from as many as 12 to 100 million receptor cells. Axons of mitral cells and tufted cells combine to form the olfactory tract.

6. The *olfactory tract* consists primarily of the axons of mitral and tufted cells. The axons of the olfactory tract lie in the olfactory sulcus on the ventral (orbital) surface of the frontal lobe, lateral to the gyrus rectus. Immediately anterior to the anterior perforated space, the olfactory tract divides into two main bundles: the lateral olfactory stria and the medial olfactory stria.

7. The anterior olfactory nucleus is formed by cells scattered along the length of the olfactory tract. The cells of this nucleus receive synaptic input by way of collateral branches of mitral and tufted cells and give rise to axons that pass through the anterior commissure to enter the olfactory tract on the contralateral side. These axons then pass into the olfactory bulb where they are thought to inhibit transmission in

mitral cells, thus participating in a negative feedback loop essential for normal olfactory function. Other anterior olfactory nucleus cells project to the septal nuclei and to the pre-optic area.

8. The olfactory tract divides posteriorly to form the medial and lateral olfactory striae, the division occurring immediately anterior to the anterior perforated space. A small intermediate stria passes through the anterior perforated space to terminate in the olfactory tubercle, one of the components of the basal forebrain.

9. Axons passing into the medial olfactory stria terminate largely in the septal nuclei. From the septal nuclei, fiber projections relay nerve impulses by way of the stria medullaris to the habenular nuclei, by way of the medial forebrain bundle to the hypothalamus, and by way of the septo-hippocampal pathway to the hippocampus.

10. Axons passing into the lateral olfactory stria terminate in the amygdaloid nuclear complex (corticomedial nucleus) and cortical areas including the lateral olfactory gyrus (primary olfactory cortex), uncus, and entorhinal cortex (olfactory association cortex [area 28]). These cortical areas are sometimes referred to as the *piriform area*. Cells in the corticomedial amygdala project axons to the hypothalamus. From the piriform area, primarily the entorhinal cortex, nerve impulses are distributed to the hippocampus by way of the perforant pathway and to the orbital cortex of the frontal lobe by way of the uncinate fasciculus.

11. (*Note*: Because much of what we know about that anatomical organization of the olfactory system is derived from studies in animals, the designation of termination sites of the fibers of the lateral olfactory stria in particular, is somewhat complicated and often confusing. Thus, the lateral olfactory gyrus, together with the lateral part of the uncus, constitutes the prepiriform cortex. The medial part of the uncus is designated as periamygdaloid cortex. Cortical areas located lateral to the uncus, extending to and along the depths of the collateral sulcus and its anterior extension, the rhinal sulcus, are referred to as *entorhinal cortex*. Collectively, these cortical areas located on the medial and ventral surface of the temporal lobe are known as the *piriform area* or lobe).

12. Odorants are presumably perceived and identified in the piriform cortex. Some evidence suggests that pleasant odors are processed in the left hemisphere while unpleasant odors are processed in the right.

13. The most common cause of impaired olfactory function is obstruction of the airway, frequently the result of an inflammatory process involving the nasal mucosa. Anosmia or hyposmia can also result

from head trauma, usually associated with forces applied in the anterior-posterior direction that shear the olfactory fila as they pass through the cribriform plate. The incidence of anosmia in head trauma is between 7% and 30%. Olfactory auras are sometimes seen in patients with epilepsy arising from lesions in the temporal lobe.

14. Some viruses, toxins, and heavy metals (aluminum) can be taken up by the olfactory system and transmitted trans-synaptically to nuclei and cortical areas within the brain.

VISUAL SYSTEM

Key Points

1. The retina is the photosensitive part of the eye. The key functional features of the retina are the *macula lutea (macula)* and the *optic disc*. The macula lutea represents the area of greatest visual acuity and the optic disc is that region of the retina that marks the attachment of the optic nerve. The optic disc is free of photoreceptors and consequently is responsible for the "blind spot" in the visual field.

2. Each retina contains approximately 130 million photoreceptor cells (124 million rods and 6 million cones). The macula is approximately 1.5 mm in diameter and contains both cones and rods. Photoreceptors in the macula respond to stimuli originating from 7 to 10 degrees of arc around the visual axis. The fovea (fovea centralis) of the retina is an area .35 mm in diameter located in the center of the macula lutea. This region is composed of exclusively cones. The cones of the fovea respond to a total visual field of approximately 1.5 to 3.0 degrees of arc around the visual axis. Visual acuity is best for images falling on the fovea centralis. This small area of the retina is used for visual tasks such as reading. The portion of the retina surrounding the macula, an area commonly referred to as the *perimacular retina*, consists almost exclusively of rods and is used for peripheral vision. Visual acuity is lowest for images activating rods in the perimacular retina. The optic disc is located to the nasal side of the macula lutea. The optic disc is approximately 1.5 mm in diameter. At the center of the optic disc is a small depression known as the *physiological cup*. The diameter of the cup is approximately 0.5 mm in healthy individuals, with the normal cup/disc ratio being 3 to 4:10.

3. Histologically, the retina consists of 10 layers. From outside to inside (superficial to deep), these layers are 1) the pigmented epithelial layer, 2) layer of rods and cones, 3) external limiting membrane, 4) outer

nuclear layer, 5) outer plexiform layer, 6) inner nuclear layer, 7) inner plexiform layer, 8) ganglion cell layer, 9) nerve fiber layer, and 10) internal limiting membrane. The *outer nuclear layer* is formed by the nuclei of rods and cones. The *inner nuclear layer* is formed by the cell bodies (nuclei) of bipolar cells. The *outer plexiform layer* lies between the outer and inner nuclear layers and is formed largely by synaptic connections involving these two types of retinal cells. The *ganglion cell layer* is formed by cell bodies of the ganglion cell. The *inner plexiform layer* lies between the inner nuclear layer and the ganglion cell layer and is formed largely by synaptic connections between bipolar cells and ganglion cells. The retina also contains a variety of other cells, most importantly horizontal and amacrine cells. These later cells are largely inhibitory in their effect.

4. *Ganglion cells* form the optic nerve, optic chiasm, and optic tract. There are approximately 1.2 million ganglion cells in each retina and therefore approximately 1.2 million axons in each optic nerve. Slightly more than half of the axons of the optic nerve subserve the foveal and macular portions of the retina. The ratio of cones to ganglion cells in the fovea is approximately 1:1, thus accounting for this area of the retina having the highest visual acuity. This ratio increases with distance from the fovea, resulting in these more peripheral areas of the retina having lower visual acuity.

5. The retina can be functionally divided into four quadrants centered around the fovea: *upper nasal, lower nasal, upper temporal,* and *lower temporal.* Light passing through the biconvex lens is bent such that light impinging on a particular retinal quadrant originates from the opposite quadrant of the visual field in terms of both side and altitude. For example, light originating in the upper temporal visual field of the right eye will act on photoreceptors in the lower nasal retinal quadrant of the right eye. Thus, we can define both visual fields and retinal quadrants.

6. The optic nerve extends from the ganglion cell body located in the retina to the anterior margin of the optic chiasm. The nerve is divided into four anatomical segments: intraocular, intraorbital, intracanalicular, and intracranial. The *intraocular* segment lies within the eye and extends from the ganglion cell body to the point where the axons pass through the lamina cribrosa. The axons of this part of the optic nerve differ in length based on the distance from the cell body to the region of the optic disc. This part of the optic nerve is unmyelinated. The *intraorbital* segment extends from the posterior surface of the globe to the anterior margin of the optic canal. This segment is approximately 25 to 30 mm in length and is myelinated. It is

approximately 8 mm longer than the distance from the posterior margin of the eye to the optic canal to permit tension-free movement of the eye. The *intracanalicular* segment lies within the optic canal to which it is tightly attached. This segment of the nerve is approximately 6 to 10 mm in length and is myelinated. The *intracranial* segment extends from the posterior opening of the optic canal to the anterior margin of the optic chiasm. This segment is myelinated and is variable in length, ranging from 10 to 25 mm, depending on the position of the optic chiasm (typical position, prefixed, or postfixed). The typical position of the optic chiasm is directly over the pituitary gland. This placement is found in approximately 80% of the population. The optic chiasm lies anterior to the pituitary (prefixed) in approximately 9% of the population and posterior to the pituitary gland in approximately 11%. Thus, the intracranial segment is correspondingly shorter or longer in individuals with a prefixed or postfixed chiasm, respectively. The position of the optic chiasm has important clinical implications in patients with expanding tumors of the pituitary gland.

7. In humans, approximately 53% of the axons in the optic nerve decussate in the optic chiasm. The axons of ganglion cells subserving nasal retinal quadrants cross the midline in the optic chasm. Axons of ganglion cells subserving temporal retinal quadrants do not decussate in the optic chiasm. Posterior to the optic chiasm, these axons form the optic tract. Axons subserving the macular quadrants are located in the posterior part of the optic chiasm.

8. Axons of the optic tract terminate in the ipsilateral lateral geniculate nucleus, pretectal nuclei, nuclei of the superior colliculus (tectum), and hypothalamus (suprachiasmatic nucleus). Fibers terminating in the lateral geniculate nucleus are part of the system involved in the process of light perception (seeing). Fibers terminating in the pretectal nuclei are part of a system involved in regulating pupil diameter and lens shape. Fibers terminating in the superior colliculus are part of a system involved in the control of eye and head position in response to visual stimuli. Fibers terminating in the hypothalamus are part of a system involved in the regulation of endocrine and hormonal release in response to changes in light intensity (brightness).

9. Cells of the lateral geniculate nucleus project axons to the ipsilateral occipital lobe, specifically to the gyri on either side of the calcarine sulcus: the *lingual* and *cuneate gyri* (primary visual cortex). Geniculocalcarine projections are retinotopically organized such that information from the lower retinal quadrants is distributed to the lingual gyrus and information from the upper retinal quadrants is distributed to the cuneate gyrus. These two gyri comprise the primary

visual (calcarine) cortex (area 17). The main function of primary visual cortex is visual perception.

10. Geniculocalcarine projections (visual radiations) occupy a large region of the subcortical white matter of the occipital, parietal, and temporal lobes. Cells located in the medial part of the lateral geniculate nucleus receive synaptic input from ganglion cells in the upper retinal quadrants of the retina and give rise to axons that terminate in the cuneate gyrus. Axons arising from these cells take a more or less direct course to the cuneate gyrus, passing posteriorly through the parietal lobe along the lateral side of the atrium of the ventricular cavity. Cells located in the lateral part of the lateral geniculate nucleus receive synaptic input from ganglion cells located in the lower quadrants of the retina and give rise to axons that terminate in the lingual gyrus. Axons arising from these cells take a more or less indirect course to the lingual gyrus, initially passing anterolaterally into the temporal lobe before turning posteriorly to pass through the parietal and occipital lobes to terminate in the lingual gyrus. These latter geniculocalcarine projections that course through the temporal lobe constitute a fiber structure known as *Meyer's loop*. Lesions involving Meyer's loop produce a contralateral homonymous superior quadrantanopsia.

11. The fovea and macular regions of the retina project to the posterior-most extent of the occipital lobe. Visual information arising from activation of the photoreceptors in the fovea reaches cells in the posterior-most regions of the primary visual cortex, an area referred to as the *occipital pole*. Information from the macular region of the retina activates cells located slightly more anteriorly in the primary visual cortex. Together, these relatively small areas of the retina project to a disproportionately large area of primary visual cortex. Slightly greater than 50% of the primary visual cortex subserves the macular and foveal portions of the retina.

12. Nerve cells of the primary visual cortex project axons to visual association cortices of the occipital lobe (Brodmann areas 18 and 19) as well as other regions of the hemisphere not primarily involved in visual experience. Projections from the primary visual cortex (area 17) to the visual association cortices (areas 18 and 19) are important in visual recognition and interpretation. Projections directed toward the medial temporal lobe are part of the "what" pathway and play a role in the identification of objects and persons. Projections directed toward the parietal lobe are part of the "where" pathway and play a role in directing movement, particularly hand movement, toward a particular

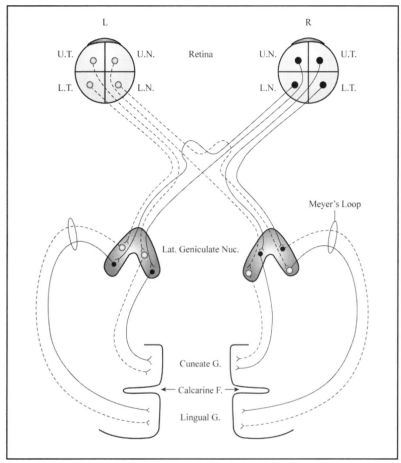

Figure 5-1: Schematic diagram of the visual pathway arising from retinal ganglion cells in each of the four retinal quadrants: U.N.=upper nasal, U.T.=upper temporal, L.N.=lower nasal, L.T.=lower temporal.

place in extra personal space. Projections to cortical areas surrounding the posterior ramus of the lateral fissure, to areas involved in certain language functions, may be important in the recognition of symbols, specifically graphemes. Lesions involving visual association cortices that spare the primary visual cortex are associated with a class of clinical findings referred to as *visual agnosia*. The visual association cortices, in turn, project axons to a number of other cortical areas and brainstem nuclei that play roles in a variety of experiential and motor functions (Figure 5-1).

13. Prechiasmatic lesions involving the visual pathway usually result in deficits involving the ipsilateral eye (*monocular* deficits). Postchiasmatic lesions usually result in visual defects involving both eyes (*binocular* deficits). Lesions involving the optic tract tend to be incongruous in form, whereas those involving the optic radiations tend to be more congruous in form. Lesions involving the occipital pole tend to affect central vision.

14. Lesions restricted to visual association cortices (areas 18 and 19) typically produce deficits of visual recognition rather than problems of light perception.

15. The visual pathway from the eye to the occipital lobe receives its arterial supply by way of branches derived from both the carotid and vertebrobasilar circulations. Structures including the eye and extending to the lateral geniculate body are perfused primarily by way of arteries derived from the internal carotid artery. Structures from the lateral geniculate to the occipital lobe are perfused primarily by way of arteries derived from the basilar artery. The visual cortices, in particular, are perfused primarily by branches of the posterior cerebral artery, specifically the calcarine artery. Cells in the region of the occipital pole are located in a "watershed" area between the posterior cerebral and middle cerebral arteries.

VISUAL REFLEXES

Key Points

1. The term *visual reflexes* commonly refers to two distinct adaptive mechanisms required for normal visual system function. The visual reflexes include the *pupillary light reflexes*, which operate to maintain proper retinal illumination in the face of changes in light intensity, and the *accommodation response* (near reflex), which operates to maintain focus on an object of interest regardless of its distance from the eye. These two physiological responses are automatic (reflex) in nature and involve both the intraocular and extraocular muscles of the eye.

2. The pupillary light reflexes operate to maintain proper retinal illumination in the face of changing light intensities. This goal is achieved by mechanisms involving the muscles of the iris, muscles that regulate the size of the pupil. Contraction of the circularly oriented constrictor muscle results in a decrease in pupil diameter, while contraction of the radially oriented dilator muscle results in an increase in pupil

size. Technically, the pupillary light reflexes include both pupillary constriction in response to increases in ambient light intensity and pupillary dilatation in response to decreases in ambient light intensity.

3. An increase in light intensity results in activation of the parasympathetic division of the autonomic nervous system and a decrease in pupil size. The afferent limb of this reflex response is formed by axons of retinal ganglion cells that constitute the optic nerves, chiasm, and optic tracts (CN II). Axons important in mediating the light reflex are collateral branches of the optic tract that terminate in the pretectal nucleus of the midbrain. The pretectal nucleus in turn projects axons to the Edinger-Westphal nucleus. The efferent limb of the light reflex is formed by preganglionic parasympathetic axons arising from nerve cell bodies located in the Edinger-Westphal nucleus and postganglionic parasympathetic axons originating from nerve cell bodies located in the ciliary ganglion located in the orbit. The preganglionic axons are thinly myelinated and are part of the oculomotor nerve (CN III). These axons are located superficially in the oculomotor nerve, and as a result, may be selectively affected in conditions in which the oculomotor nerve is compressed at some point along its course. Such compression might occur in association with uncal herniation or in patients with aneurysms of the posterior communication artery. The postganglionic axons arise from the ciliary ganglion, are unmyelinated, and form the short ciliary nerve. The pretectal nuclei are interconnected across the midline by way of short interneurons, as are the Edinger-Westphal nuclei of the two sides. As a result, light-activated nerve impulses impinging on cells on one side of the brainstem can activate responses in both eyes (Figure 5-2).

4. A decrease in light intensity results in an increase in pupil size. This particular response is likely mediated by two mechanisms: 1) reduced activation of photoreceptors in the eye and thus reduced impulse transmission in the optic nerves, and 2) increased activation of the sympathetic division of the autonomic nervous system. The afferent limb of this reflex response is formed by axons of retinal ganglion cells that constitute the optic nerves, chiasm, and optic tracts (CN II). Axons important in mediating pupillary dilatation are collateral branches of the optic tract that terminate in the midbrain reticular formation and hypothalamus. Cells in these two brain regions are the origin of axons that descend to upper thoracic levels of the spinal cord, where they terminate on preganglionic sympathetic cells of the intermediolateral nucleus (sometimes referred to as the ciliospinal nucleus). These latter cells give rise to thinly myelinated axons that

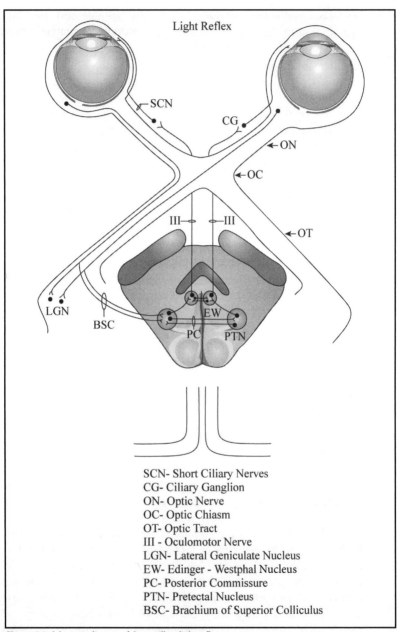

SCN- Short Ciliary Nerves
CG- Ciliary Ganglion
ON- Optic Nerve
OC- Optic Chiasm
OT- Optic Tract
III - Oculomotor Nerve
LGN- Lateral Geniculate Nucleus
EW- Edinger - Westphal Nucleus
PC- Posterior Commissure
PTN- Pretectal Nucleus
BSC- Brachium of Superior Colliculus

Figure 5-2: Schematic diagram of the pupillary light reflex.

ascend in the sympathetic chain to upper cervical vertebral levels (C1-C4), where they terminate on postganglionic sympathetic nerve cells, forming the superior cervical ganglion. Axons of postganglionic sympathetic cells pass into the skull in the perivascular connective tissue of the internal carotid artery. While passing through the cavernous sinus, these fibers likely shift position to become incorporated into the ophthalmic nerve (ophthalmic division of the trigeminal nerve) and as part of this nerve, enter the orbit by way of the superior orbital fissure. Within the orbit, these fibers split from the ophthalmic nerve as the long ciliary nerve, which innervates the dilator muscles of the iris. Pupillary dilatation in response to reduced light intensity is thus mediated by the sympathetic division of the autonomic nervous system.

5. Clinically, the pupillary light reflex refers to pupillary constriction in response to increased retinal illumination. This reflex is elicited and evaluated in the clinical setting with the aid of a penlight or an ophthalmologic light of greater intensity. The normal response to illuminating one eye is bilateral pupillary constriction. The response observed in the illuminated eye is referred to as the *direct light reflex*. The response observed in the nonilluminated eye is referred to as the *indirect (consensual) light reflex*. Characteristics of the elicited response to be noted include response latency and magnitude. The briskness of the light reflexes decreases with age.

6. The accommodation response (near reflex) operates to help maintain visual acuity when viewing objects at short distances from the eye (within approximately 35 cm or 14 in). The near reflex consists of three components: ocular adduction, pupillary constriction, and accommodation of the lens. *Ocular adduction* results from contraction of the medial rectus muscle, *pupillary constriction* occurs in response to contraction of the pupillary constrictor muscle, and *accommodation of the lens* results from contraction of the ciliary muscle, a muscle whose fibers form the ciliary body. (Accommodation of the lens refers to the process whereby the shape of the lens is changed to reduce the focal length of the optic system. During accommodation, the focal length of the lens becomes shorter, thereby allowing the viewer to focus more clearly on near objects, typically at distances of 35 cm or less in front of the eye. The process involves contraction of the circularly-oriented ciliary muscle, which reduces tension on the radially-oriented zonular fibers attached to the lens. Reduced tension causes the lens to become slightly more spherical in shape, which in turn increases the convexity of the anterior and posterior surfaces of the lens. The greater the convexity of the anterior and

posterior surfaces of the lens, the greater the lens will "bend" light passing through it.) The medial rectus is innervated by alpha motor neurons located in the oculomotor nucleus with axons that form the bulk of the oculomotor nerve. The pupillary constrictor and ciliary muscles are innervated by cells of the autonomic nervous system. The preganglionic cell body is located in the Edinger-Westphal nucleus, a part of the oculomotor complex. The axons of these cells are part of the oculomotor nerve. The postganglionic cell body is located in the ciliary ganglion. The axons of the postganglionic cells form the short ciliary nerve. Ninety-five to 97% of the cells of the ciliary ganglion innervate the ciliary muscle, with the remaining cells providing innervation to the constrictor muscle of the pupil (Figure 5-3).

7. The neural pathway for the accommodation reflex is somewhat more complicated than that mediating the pupillary light reflex, and involves the primary visual cortex (area 17) of the occipital lobe. In brief, retinal ganglion cells (specifically those responding to stimulation of the fovea) project to the lateral geniculate nuclei, which in turn project by way of the visual radiations (geniculo-calcarine projections) to the primary visual cortex (area 17) of the occipital lobe (lingual and cuneate gyri). Cells in the primary visual cortex (area 17) project axons to visual association cortices (areas 18 and 19), which in turn project axons to the superior colliculus and prefrontal eye fields. The superior colliculus and prefrontal eye fields give rise to axons that project to and terminate in the oculomotor nucleus (medial rectus subnucleus) and the Edinger-Westphal nucleus. These two nuclei then give rise to axons that innervate structures that result in ocular adduction, pupillary constriction, and accommodation of the lens.

8. Clinically, the accommodation reflex is evaluated by observing the degree to which the pupils constrict and the eyes adduct when the subject is asked to shift gaze from a distant object to a near object or when the subject is asked to maintain visual fixation on an object (such as the tip of the examiner's finger) as it is moved from a distance toward the subject's nose. Accommodation of the lens, which is necessary to keep the finger in focus as it approaches the nose, is not visible to the examiner.

9. Lesions or disease processes that interrupt or impair nerve impulse transmission in the optic nerve affect the direct light reflex in the involved eye and the indirect light reflex in the uninvolved eye. Such patients demonstrate a *relative afferent pupillary defect* (RAPD) on the involved side, sometimes referred to as a *Marcus-Gunn pupil*. When performing the swinging flashlight test in such patients, the indirect response in the involved eye is greater than the direct response. That

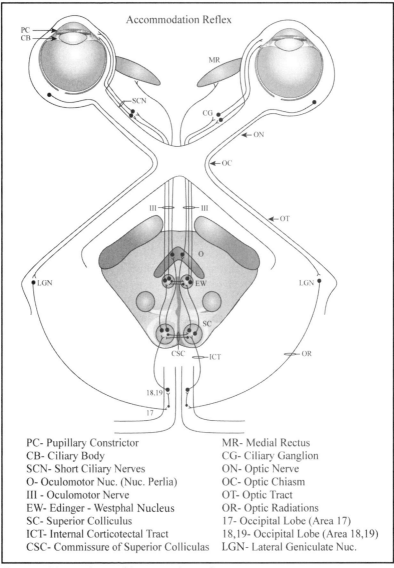

Figure 5-3: Schematic diagram of the accommodation reflex.

is, when the light source is rapidly moved from the intact eye to the involved eye, the pupil in the involved eye will be observed to dilate, a phenomenon sometimes referred to as a *paradoxical response*. Also, in individuals with lesions involving the optic nerve, pupillary constriction during accommodation (near vision) remains intact even though pupillary constriction in response to direct light stimulation is impaired. Lesions involving the optic tract may result in subtle, difficult-to-detect changes in the light reflex. Lesions affecting the visual radiations leave the light reflexes intact.

OCULAR MOTOR SYSTEM —OCULAR MUSCLES AND MOVEMENTS

Key Points

1. The main function of the extraocular muscles is to move and position the eye in order to bring an object of interest onto the macula lutea of the retina.

2. Eye movements are rotatory in nature, occurring around three perpendicular axes (Fick's axes) that pass through the center of the eye. Eye movements are named with reference to the direction the pupil moves relative to the position of primary gaze (eyes looking straight ahead). Supraduction (elevation) and subduction (depression) occur around a lateral-horizontal axis (X axis). Abduction and adduction occur around a vertical axis (Z axis). Incycloduction (intorsion) and excycloduction (extorsion) occur around an anterior-posterior axis (Y axis).

3. Eye movements are the result of the coordinated action of six muscles acting on each eye: the superior, inferior, medial, and lateral rectus muscles and the superior and inferior oblique muscles. The four rectus muscles originate from a common tendinous ring near the apex of the orbit and extend anteriorly along their respective sides of the eye. The rectus muscles insert into the eye anterior to Listing's plane, a functional landmark that divides the eye into anterior and posterior halves. The superior oblique muscle also originates from the common tendinous ring and passes anteriorly toward the superomedial margin of the orbit, where its tendon passes through a small opening in the periosteum (trochlea) before passing posterolaterally on the superior surface of the eye to insert posterior to Listing's plane. The inferior oblique is a short muscle that originates from the inferomedial aspect of the orbit and passes posterolaterally on the inferior surface of the eye to insert posterior to Listing's plane.

4. Two muscles (lateral and medial rectus) move the eye around only one axis (vertical axis). The remaining four muscles, because of their course and attachment to the eye, move the eye with relatively different efficiencies around all three axes. The most efficient action

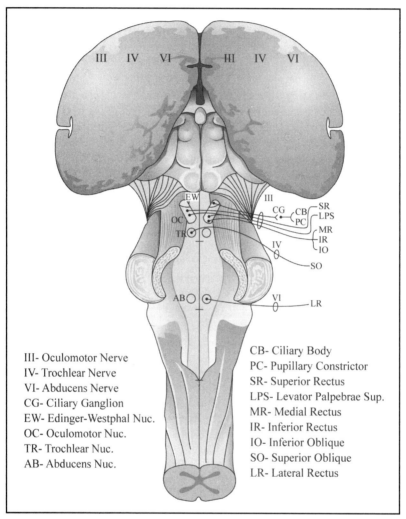

Figure 5-4: Lower motor innervation of the extraocular muscles and levator palpebrae superioris.

produced by contraction of each muscle, starting from the position of primary gaze, is referred to as the *primary action*. The less efficient actions are referred to as the *secondary* and *tertiary actions*. From a functional perspective, it is important to understand the primary and secondary actions of each extraocular muscle.

5. The lateral rectus is innervated by the abducens nerve (Figure 5-4). The abducens nucleus lies in the caudal pons, near the midline. The

axons course ventrally through the pontine tegmentum to exit the brainstem at the level of the ponto-medullary junction. They then course anteriorly through the prepontine cistern, passing below the petroclinoid ligament to reach the posterior wall of the cavernous sinus. The nerve enters the cavernous sinus by passing through a small opening (Dorello's canal). Within the cavernous sinus, the abducens nerve courses anteriorly, lying lateral to the internal carotid artery. The nerve enters the orbit through the superior orbital fissure, passes through the common tendinous ring, and courses anteriorly, lying on the deep surface of the lateral rectus muscle. The lateral rectus muscle is innervated by nerve cells located in the ipsilateral abducens nucleus.

6. The superior oblique is innervated by the trochlear nerve. The trochlear nucleus lies in the caudal half of the midbrain at the level of the inferior colliculus, near the anterior margin of the periaqueductal gray. The axons of these cells course dorsolaterally around the periaqueductal gray and cross the midline in the inferior medullary velum before exiting the brainstem at the inferior margin of the inferior colliculus. The nerve passes anteriorly through the quadrigeminal and crural cisterns and enters the lateral wall of the cavernous sinus, where it lies below the fibers of the oculomotor nerve and above the fibers of the ophthalmic nerve. The nerve courses anteriorly through the lateral wall of the cavernous sinus and enters the orbit by way of the superior orbital fissure. Within the orbit, the axons pass above the common tendinous ring, outside the muscle cone, and come to lie on the deep surface of the superior oblique muscle. The superior oblique is innervated by nerve cells located in the contralateral trochlear nucleus.

7. The superior rectus, medial rectus, inferior rectus, and inferior oblique are all innervated by the oculomotor nerve, as is the levator palpebrae superioris. The oculomotor nucleus lies in the rostral half of the midbrain at the level of the superior colliculus. The oculomotor nucleus is composed of six subnuclei, four of which contain cells that innervate the four muscles mentioned above, another of which innervates the levator palpebrae superioris, and the last of which is the Edinger-Westphal nucleus, a collection of preganglionic parasympathetic cells that give rise to axons that terminate in the ciliary ganglion. The axons of the cells of the oculomotor nucleus course ventrally through the mesencephalic tegmentum, passing through the red nucleus and medial part of the cerebral peduncle to emerge from the brainstem at the level of the interpeduncular fossa. The axons course

anteriorly through the interpeduncular cistern, passing between the posterior cerebral artery and the superior cerebellar artery. The nerve courses above the petroclinoid ligament to enter the lateral wall of the cavernous sinus, where it lies above the fibers of the trochlear nerve. The nerve passes anteriorly in the lateral wall of the sinus and passes into the orbit through the superior orbital fissure. In the region of the superior orbital fissure, the nerve divides into superior and inferior branches, both of which pass anteriorly through the common tendinous ring. The superior branch carries axons that innervate the superior rectus and levator palpebrae superioris and the inferior branch carries axons that innervate the medial rectus, inferior rectus, and inferior oblique. (*Note:* The inferior branch also carries preganglionic parasympathetic axons destined for the ciliary ganglion.)

8. The position of primary gaze is characterized by the eye in the upright head looking straight ahead. All six extraocular muscles are tonically active when the eye is in the position of primary gaze, the position being maintained as a result of offsetting actions of agonist and antagonist muscles. The efficient movement of the eye is the result of changes in the frequency of nerve impulses delivered to all six eye muscles operating on that eye. These alterations in nerve cell activity operate in compliance with *Sherrington's law* (law of reciprocal innervation), which fundamentally states that as a particular muscle is excited to produce a desired movement, its antagonist(s) is reciprocally inhibited. For example, to abduct the right eye, the right lateral rectus must contract and the right medial rectus must relax. Stated differently, to abduct the right eye, nerve cells in the right abducens nucleus must be excited (increase their firing frequency) and cells in the right oculomotor nucleus must be inhibited (decrease their firing frequency).

9. The key to understanding normal and abnormal ocular motor function requires an understanding of 1) the precise origin and insertion of each extraocular muscle, 2) the innervation of each muscle, 3) the primary and secondary action(s) of each muscle, and 4) the muscle(s) involved in moving the eye in each of the cardinal directions (Figure 5-5).

10. Lesions involving the extraocular nuclei or their axons typically result in displacement of the eye (and visual axis of that eye) away from the position of primary gaze. The position at rest in the affected eye will be determined by the activity of the unaffected muscles working in the absence of the affected muscle. When looking at the two eyes together in an individual so affected who is not compensating for the

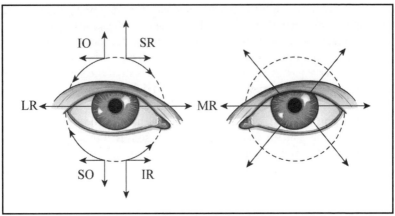

Figure 5-5: Actions of individual extraocular muscles. The length of the arrows indicates the relative strength of the different actions of each muscle in moving the eye starting from the position of primary gaze.

abnormality by repositioning the head, the visual axes of the two eyes will be seen to be not parallel—a condition referred to as *strabismus*. Malalignment of the visual axes of the two eyes present when the subject is attempting to fixate on a target of interest with both eyes open is referred to as *heterotropia,* or more commonly, *tropia.* Tropias are named according to the direction of displacement of the pupil in the involved eye. Patients with acute tropia commonly complain of diplopia. Patients with tropia of longer duration may learn to ignore information from one eye.

11. Patients demonstrating tropia frequently (but not always) compensate by repositioning the head, using the intact muscles of the unaffected eye to reposition that eye so that the visual axes of the two eyes will be parallel.

12. Individual eye muscles can be tested by placing the eye in a position where the pull of the muscle to be tested is perpendicular to a single axis of rotation (Figures 5-6 and 5-7).

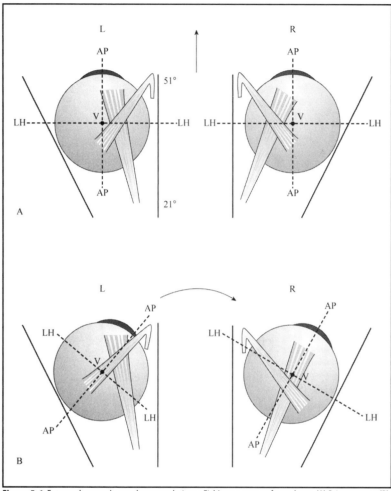

Figure 5-6: Extraocular muscle attachments relative to Fick's axes as seen from above. (A) Primary gaze, (B) right gaze shift. (Note that the relative efficiency of each muscle in producing a particular movement varies with the position of the eye.) LH=lateral-horizontal axis, AP=anterior-posterior axis.

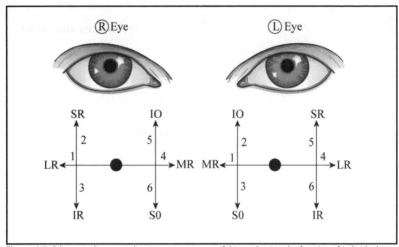

Figure 5-7: Schematic diagram indicating movements useful in evaluating the function of individual eye muscles.

OCULAR MOTOR SYSTEM— BINOCULAR MECHANISMS

Key Points

1. In humans, two-thirds of the visual field is projected onto the retina of both eyes. One important function of the ocular motor system, therefore, is to control eye movements and position each eye so that an object of interest projects to corresponding points on each retina and is thus perceived as only a single object. The neural systems designed to achieve these goals operate both automatically (reflexively) and volitionally.

2. The main functions of the ocular motor system are gaze shifting and gaze holding. (*Note*: The term *gaze* refers to movement involving both eyes.) *Gaze shifting* refers to the ability to move both eyes to place a new or different image on the macula of both retinae. Gaze shifting can be stimulus driven (automatic/reflex) or nonstimulus driven (voluntary). *Gaze holding* refers to the ability to maintain binocular fixation on an object of interest when the head is moving, when the object of interest is moving, or when both are moving.

3. Two types of eye movements are necessary to maintain image fixation on the fovea of both eyes: version movements and vergence movements. In *version movements,* the visual axes of the two eyes remain parallel as the eyes move. Version movements are sometimes described as *gaze shifts* (right gaze shift, left gaze shift, upward gaze shift, and downward gaze shift). Version movements are used to maintain binocular fixation on moving or relatively moving objects that are located at distances of greater than approximately 35 cm (14 in). *Vergence movements* occur when the visual axes of the two eyes do not remain parallel as the eyes move. Two types of vergence movements are described: convergence and divergence. *Convergence* (convergent movement) refers to bilateral ocular adduction, the type of eye movements needed to maintain binocular fixation on an object as it moves toward the head, particularly within 14 inches of the face. Ocular convergence is part of the accommodation reflex. *Divergence* (divergent movement) refers to bilateral ocular abduction. Humans can only abduct the eyes to the position of primary gaze (ie, a position in which the visual axes of the two eyes are parallel). Divergence occurs in humans only when attempting to maintain fixation on an object moving away from the face, starting within a distance of about 14 inches. Vergence movements are used to maintain binocular fixation on objects that are moving either toward or away from the face, particularly within a distance of approximately 14 inches.

4. Version and vergence eye movements are coordinated by way of specific nuclei in the brainstem referred to as *gaze centers.* The role of the gaze centers is to project (distribute) the appropriate excitatory and inhibitory influences to the extraocular nuclei (oculomotor, trochlear, and abducens) so as to produce the intended movement needed to maintain binocular fixation. Two main gaze centers are described, a *pontine gaze center* and a *mesencephalic gaze center.* A third group of cells, the nucleus prepositus, participates in the coordination of eye movements in response to changes in head position (Figure 5-8).

5. The pontine gaze center is represented by a group of cells located in the *paramedian pontine reticular formation* (PPRF) in the region of the abducens nucleus. These cells are sometimes referred to as forming the paraabducens nucleus. These cells, when stimulated, excite the abducens nucleus on the ipsilateral side and the oculomotor nucleus (medial rectus subnucleus) on the contralateral side. The result is conjugate gaze shift the ipsilateral side. The PPRF is therefore considered to be a center for horizontal gaze. Cells of the paraabducens nucleus that excite the cells of the contralateral oculomotor nucleus do so by way of axons that course rostrally as part of the contralateral medial

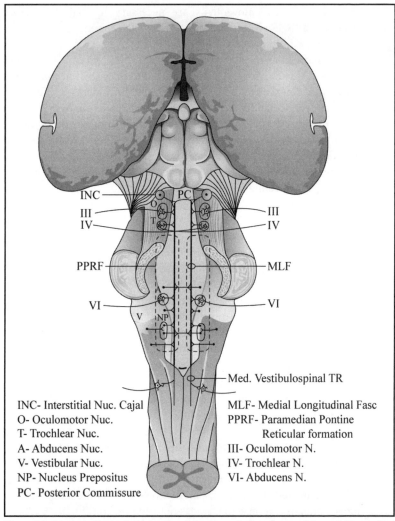

INC
III
IV
PPRF
VI
PC
III
IV
MLF
VI
O
T
V
NP
Med. Vestibulospinal TR

INC- Interstitial Nuc. Cajal
O- Oculomotor Nuc.
T- Trochlear Nuc.
A- Abducens Nuc.
V- Vestibular Nuc.
NP- Nucleus Prepositus
PC- Posterior Commissure

MLF- Medial Longitudinal Fasc
PPRF- Paramedian Pontine
        Reticular formation
III- Oculomotor N.
IV- Trochlear N.
VI- Abducens N.

Figure 5-8: Schematic diagram indicating the origin and termination of axons of the medial longitudinal fasciculus (MLF).

longitudinal fasciculus. Nuclear lesions involving the PPRF result in paresis of ipsilateral gaze shift (inability to shift gaze to the side of the lesion) (Figure 5-9).

6. The midbrain gaze center is represented by two small nuclei located along the lateral margin of the periaqueductal gray at the level of the oculomotor nucleus. These nuclei are the *rostral interstitial nucleus of*

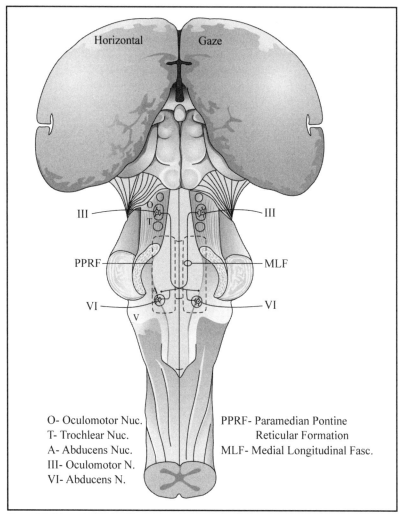

Horizontal   Gaze

III — — III

PPRF — — MLF

VI — — VI

O- Oculomotor Nuc.
T- Trochlear Nuc.
A- Abducens Nuc.
III- Oculomotor N.
VI- Abducens N.

PPRF- Paramedian Pontine
        Reticular Formation
MLF- Medial Longitudinal Fasc.

Figure 5-9: Schematic diagram of brainstem pathways involved in horizontal gaze shift.

the medial longitudinal fasciculus (riMLF) and the *interstitial nucleus of Cajal* (INC). When stimulated, the riMLF results in vertical gaze shifts. (The INC is thought to be involved in the maintenance of an eccentric eye position following vertical gaze shift.) The axons of the cells of the midbrain gaze centers project bilaterally to the oculomotor and trochlear nuclei by way of the MLF, where they influence cells that innervate muscles involved in vertical eye movements. Lesions

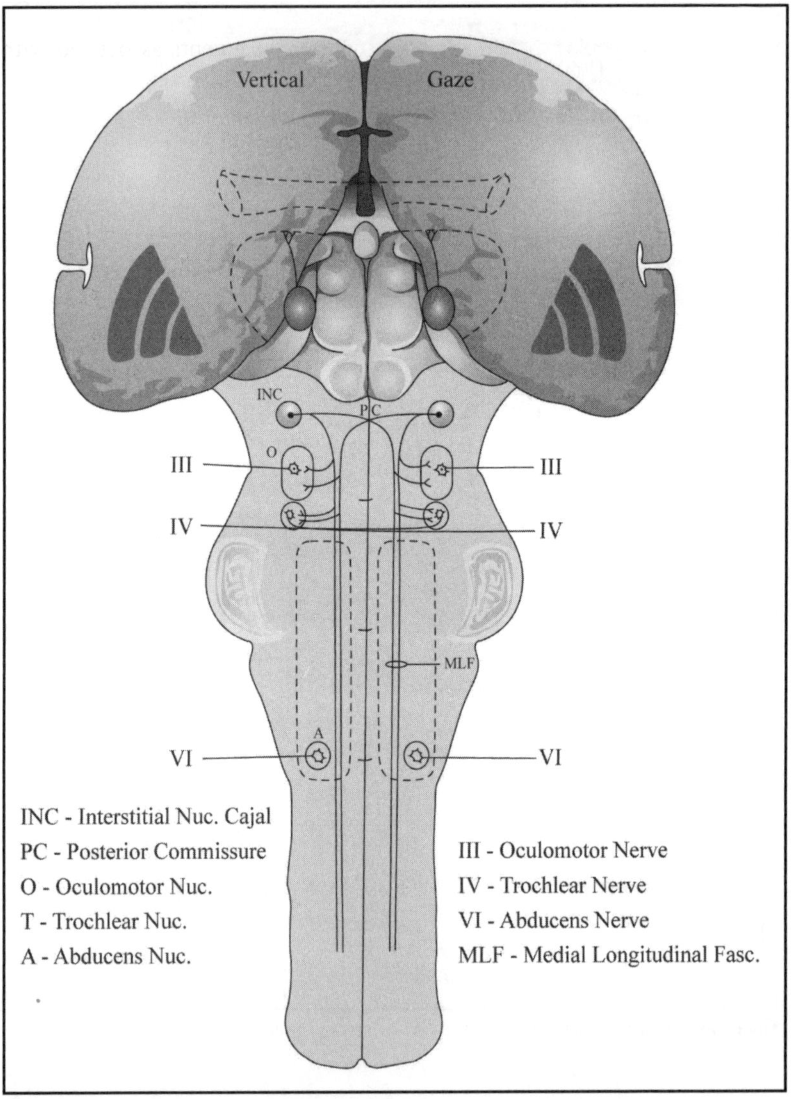

Figure 5-10: Schematic diagram of brainstem pathways involved in vertical gaze shifts.

that affect the midbrain gaze centers (usually compressive in nature) impair vertical (usually upward) eye movements (Figure 5-10).

7. The nucleus prepositus located medial to the vestibular nuclei in the rostral pons is sometimes considered to be a gaze center. This nucleus receives projections from the vestibular nuclei and projects axons

to all three ocular motor nuclei by way of the MLF. This nucleus is thought to play a role in mediating eye movements associated with the vestibulo-ocular reflexes.

8. The brainstem gaze centers project appropriate excitatory and inhibitory impulses to the extraocular nuclei in accordance with the predictions of Hering's law (law of yoked muscles). *Hering's law* states that the muscles involved in conjugate eye movements are reciprocally excited or inhibited. For example, when the right lateral rectus is excited to abduct the right eye as part of right gaze shift, the left medial rectus is simultaneously excited to produce adduction of the left eye. Likewise, when the right medial rectus is inhibited to facilitate abduction of the right eye during right gaze shift, the left lateral rectus is inhibited to facilitate adduction of the left eye. Hering's law describes the effect of nerve impulses delivered simultaneously to both eyes.

9. Injuries involving the ocular motor nerves generally result in strabismus. Strabismus that is evident when both eyes are open and fixating (manifest strabismus) is referred to as tropia (heterotropia). Tropias are named according to the position of the nonfixating eye. The evaluation of strabismus requires an understanding of the mechanisms and principles responsible for specific clinical findings observed in patients who present with tropia. One such mechanism is the mechanism responsible for the clinical finding of primary and secondary deviation. The ocular manifestations of primary and secondary deviation reflect the application of Hering's law and Sherrington's law. In an individual with manifest tropia (meaning that when viewing with both eyes, the visual axes of the two eyes are not parallel) resulting from damage to a particular cranial nerve, the angle subtended by the visual axes will be different when the individual is permitted to fixate with only one eye at a time. The angle subtended by the visual axes when the uninvolved eye is fixating is referred to as the *primary* (1 degree) deviation and the angle subtended by the visual axes when the involved eye is fixating is referred to as the *secondary* (2 degrees). In an individual with tropia resulting from lesions involving one of the ocular motor nerves, the secondary deviation will be greater than the primary deviation. This finding reflects the application of Hering's law and can be demonstrated by means of the single cover test or the cover-uncover test. Other testing methods, including red glass testing and the corneal light reflection test, can be helpful in evaluating individuals with tropia.

10. The clinical designation of tropia as either comitant or incomitant is also helpful in the evaluation of patients presenting with tropia.

Comitant tropia refers to a malalignment of the visual axes in which the angle subtended by the two visual axes does not change with gaze shift. Comitant tropia is suggestive of central nervous system (CNS) lesions involving corticonuclear upper motor neurons. Individuals with comitant tropia typically do not complain of diplopia. Such abnormalities may be congenital in nature. *Incomitant tropia* refers to a malalignment of the visual axes in which the angle subtended by the two visual axes does change with gaze shift. Incomitant tropia is suggestive of lesions involving the cells of the extraocular nuclei or their axons. Individuals with incomitant tropia may report diplopia, particularly when the eyes are moved into positions requiring the action of the affected muscle(s). Patients may compensate by holding their head in positions that minimize the needs for the weak muscle(s). Lesions that result in incomitant tropia are typically acquired in nature.

11. *Phoria* (heterophoria) refers to a type of ocular motor abnormality characterized by malalignment of the visual axes when fixation is blocked in one eye. Individuals with phoria are able to maintain binocular fixation when both eyes are open and viewing, but demonstrate ocular deviation in a particular direction when one eye is covered. Phorias are named by the direction of deviation of the eye when fixation is prevented in that eye (when the eye is covered with an occluder). Phoria may "break down", resulting in the development of a tropia. Phorias are commonly identified by means of the alternate cover test.

OCULAR MOTOR SYSTEM— VOLITIONAL AND PURSUIT MOVEMENTS

Key Points

1. Two types of eye movements are initiated in the cerebral cortex. These movements are commonly referred to as saccades and pursuit eye movements. *Saccades* are relatively quick, conjugate eye movements initiated by cells in the frontal lobe. Voluntary eye movements are one form of saccadic eye movements. *Pursuit eye movements* are relatively slow eye movements that are initiated by cells in the parieto-occipital cortex. Pursuit eye movements are sometimes referred to as *tracking* eye movements.

2. Voluntary saccades are intended to position or move the eyes so that the individual can look at and focus on a particular object of interest

at will. Functionally, the cortical cells involved in these so-called *volitional* eye movements are located anterior to the precentral sulcus in the middle frontal gyrus in an area referred to as the *frontal (prefrontal) eye fields* (Brodmann area 8). Axons arising from these cells pass inferiorly through the corona radiata and into the posterior part of the anterior limb of the internal capsule. The axons continue caudally through the middle region of the cerebral peduncle before entering the pons, where they terminate. In the midbrain, these fibers give rise to collateral branches that terminate in the oculomotor and trochlear nuclei and the midbrain gaze centers. In the pons, these axons are part of the longitudinal pontine bundles and terminate bilaterally in the pontine gaze center of the PPRF. (*Note:* At the level of the rostral midbrain, a collateral descending pathway arises from these fibers. This pathway is located in a more dorsal position, passing through the central regions of the mesencephalic and pontine reticular formation. These fibers terminate predominantly in the pontine gaze center and form a pathway referred to as the *aberrant corticonuclear (corticobulbar) tract.*)

3. Activation of the cells of the prefrontal eye fields from other regions of the cerebral cortex results in conjugate deviation of the eyes to the contralateral side (contralateral gaze shift). Voluntary eye movements are produced by activation of the frontal eye fields by cells located more anteriorly in the frontal lobe. (*Note:* These cells can also be activated by sensory system association cells as part of neural systems that produce eye movements in response to auditory, tactile, olfactory, and certain types of visual stimuli.) Volitional vertical gaze shifts result from bilateral activation of the frontal eye fields (Figure 5-11).

4. Destructive lesions involving the frontal eye fields are associated with inability to shift gaze to the contralateral side. In the acute phase of certain brain disorders such as stroke, patients may present with tonic deviation of the eyes to the ipsilateral side (side of the infarction). Focal conditions, such as those resulting in partial seizures affecting the frontal eye fields, may be associated with deviation of the eyes to the contralateral side (Figure 5-12).

5. Pursuit eye movements (visual pursuit or tracking movements) are intended to maintain fixation on moving objects. This system operates both when the head is stationary and when it is moving. (*Note:* When the head is moving, the vestibular nuclei also act on the extraocular nuclei and the pursuit mechanisms will be required to adapt accordingly.) Functionally, the cortical cells involved in pursuit movements are located in the occipital and parietal lobes, in the

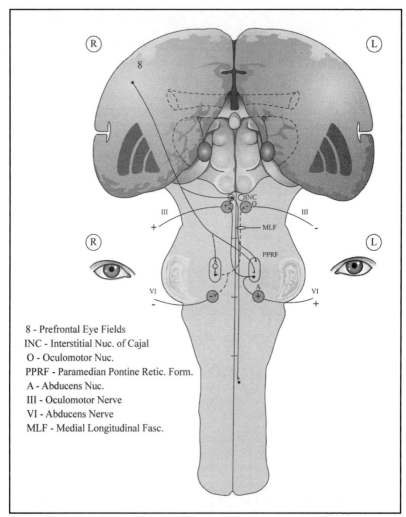

Figure 5-11: Schematic diagram of the pathway for voluntary eye movements (coronal view).

8 - Prefrontal Eye Fields
INC - Interstitial Nuc. of Cajal
O - Oculomotor Nuc.
PPRF - Paramedian Pontine Retic. Form.
A - Abducens Nuc.
III - Oculomotor Nerve
VI - Abducens Nerve
MLF - Medial Longitudinal Fasc.

visual association cortices (Brodmann areas 18 and 19). These cells are activated mainly by primary visual cortex cells related to photoreceptors located in the macula and fovea of the retina. Axons arising from these cells pass inferiorly through the corona radiata to terminate in the mesencephalic and pontine gaze centers, with collateral branches terminating in the nucleus of the superior colliculus. The cells of the

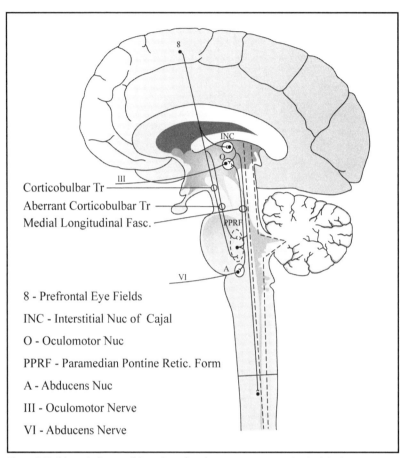

Figure 5-12: Schematic diagram of the pathway for voluntary eye movements (sagittal view).

superior colliculus in turn project axons to the mesencephalic and pontine gaze centers and to all three extraocular nuclei. (*Note*: Other cells of the visual association cortex project axons anteriorly by way of the superior longitudinal fasciculus to terminate in the frontal eye fields. This projection pathway may play a role in the initial saccade to fixate on an object of interest [visual grasp] located in the temporal, monocular part of the visual field; Figure 5-13.)

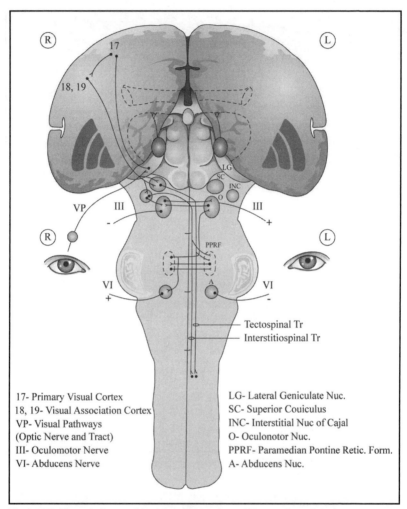

Figure 5-13: Schematic diagram of the pathway for pursuit eye movements (coronal view).

6. Destructive lesions involving the visual association cortices or the underlying white matter most commonly result in visual field defects and visual agnosia, which may make it difficult to evaluate visual pursuit function. Evidence suggests that patients with lesions involving the posterior parieto-occipital areas have difficulty pursuing objects moving from the midline to the ipsilateral side (Figure 5-14).

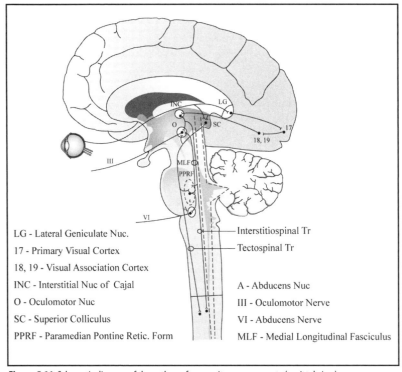

LG - Lateral Geniculate Nuc.
17 - Primary Visual Cortex
18, 19 - Visual Association Cortex
INC - Interstitial Nuc of Cajal
O - Oculomotor Nuc
SC - Superior Colliculus
PPRF - Paramedian Pontine Retic. Form

Interstitiospinal Tr
Tectospinal Tr

A - Abducens Nuc
III - Oculomotor Nerve
VI - Abducens Nerve
MLF - Medial Longitudinal Fasciculus

Figure 5-14: Schematic diagram of the pathway for pursuit eye movements (sagittal view).

TRIGEMINAL NERVE

Key Points

1. The main functions of the trigeminal nerve are to provide sensory innervation to the face and meninges of the anterior and middle cranial fossa and motor innervation to the muscles of mastication. It also serves as the afferent limb of the corneal reflex and the afferent and efferent limbs of the masseter reflex.

2. The trigeminal nerve emerges from the ventrolateral aspect of the pons by way of two roots: a large sensory root (portio major) and a smaller motor root (portio minor). The afferent cell bodies of the sensory root form the trigeminal ganglion, sometimes referred to as the *semilunar* or *Gasserian ganglion*. The ganglion lies in Meckel's cave, immediately superior to foramen ovale in the middle cranial fossa.

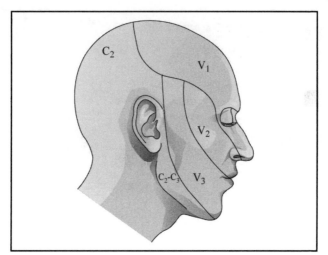

Figure 5-15: Schematic diagram indicating the cutaneous distribution of the ophthalmic (V1), maxillary (V2), and mandibular (V3) divisions of the trigeminal nerve.

The three major branches of the trigeminal nerve: *ophthalmic* (V1), *maxillary* (V2), and *mandibular* (V3) exit the middle cranial fossa by way of the superior orbital fissure, foramen rotundum, and foramen ovale, respectively.

3. The ophthalmic nerve provides sensory innervation to the forehead, upper eyelid, anterior half of the scalp, the eye including the cornea, and the frontal and ethmoidal sinuses. The maxillary nerve provides sensory innervation to the skin over the maxilla and upper lip, mucous lining of the nasal cavity, nasopharynx and maxillary sinus, the hard and soft palate, and the maxillary teeth and gingiva. The mandibular nerve provides sensory innervation to the skin over the mandible (excluding the angle), anterior two-thirds of the tongue and surrounding oral mucosa, and the mandibular teeth and gingiva. All three divisions give rise to meningeal branches that provide sensory innervation to the intracranial meninges (Figure 5-15).

4. The central processes of trigeminal ganglion cells enter the brainstem at the level of the rostral part of the pons. Upon entry, the axons divide into two components: a descending component, composed of predominantly unmyelinated and thinly myelinated axons that extends caudally to upper cervical segments of the spinal cord (C1-C3), and a component composed of predominantly myelinated axons that terminates in nuclei at the level of entry in the rostral pons. The descending axons form a pathway known as the *spinal trigeminal tract*

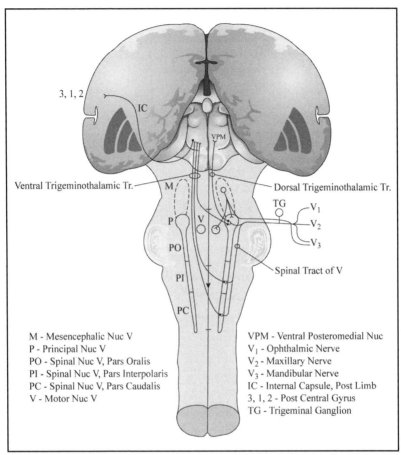

Figure 5-16: Schematic diagram of the central connections of the trigeminal nerve and spinal trigeminal nuclei.

(spinal tract of V). The axons of the spinal trigeminal tract terminate in the spinal trigeminal nucleus (spinal nucleus of V), a small, multi-segmental nucleus extending from the rostral pons to upper cervical cord levels and in various nuclei of pontine and medullary reticular formation. The tract lies along the lateral edge of the spinal trigeminal nucleus throughout the length of the pons and medulla oblongata. The axons of the spinal trigeminal tract are somatotopically organized with those derived from the ophthalmic nerve lying ventral within the tract and those derived from the mandibular nerve lying more dorsally (Figure 5-16).

5. The spinal trigeminal nucleus is divided into three anatomically distinct regions defined by their anatomical location: pars caudalis, extending from upper cervical spinal cord levels to the level of the obex; pars interpolaris, extending from the obex to the level of the abducens nucleus; and pars oralis, extending from the abducens nucleus to the principal nucleus of the trigeminal nerve. Pars caudalis, sometimes referred to as *nucleus caudalis*, receives synaptic input from large numbers of unmyelinated and thinly myelinated axons, and is thus the part of the spinal trigeminal nucleus that transmits nociceptive impulses to more rostral levels of the nervous system. Histologically, pars caudalis consists of two parts: pars gelatinosa and pars magnocellularis, which represent the rostral continuation of the substantia gelatinosa and nucleus proprius of the spinal cord, respectively. Pars interpolaris and pars oralis are comparatively small and histologically uniform.

6. The principal nucleus of the trigeminal nerve, sometimes referred to as the *chief sensory nucleus of V* or the *main sensory nucleus of V*, lies at the rostral end of the spinal trigeminal nucleus, in the rostral pons, at the level where the axons of the trigeminal nerve enter the brainstem. The principal nucleus of the trigeminal nerve receives synaptic input from heavily myelinated axons transmitting nerve impulses arising from the activation of low threshold (non-nociceptive) receptors.

7. The most heavily myelinated afferent axons in the trigeminal nerve transmit nerve impulses to the brainstem from muscle spindles located predominantly in the muscles of mastication. The cell bodies of these afferent axons are located, not in the trigeminal ganglion as might be expected, but rather within the midbrain along the lateral aspect of the periaqueductal gray in a structure referred to as the *mesencephalic nucleus of the trigeminal nerve* (mesencephalic nucleus of V). The cell bodies of this nucleus are pseudounipolar in shape (like other neural crest-derived afferent cells), with a peripheral process that extends to a receptor (muscle spindle) in the periphery and a central process that makes synaptic contact with alpha motor neurons and association cells (again, like other neural crest derived afferent cells) within the CNS. The cells of the mesencephalic nucleus of the trigeminal nerve, by virtue of their central connections, are likely to play a role in mediating muscle stretch reflexes, specifically the masseter reflex (jaw jerk) and proprioceptive experiences from the mouth.

8. Axons of cells of the spinal trigeminal nucleus cross the midline near their origin and assemble near the dorsal aspect of the medial lemniscus in the pons, forming the ventral trigeminothalamic tract. These

axons lie along the medial edge of the medial lemniscus at the level of the midbrain and terminate in the ventral posteromedial nucleus of the thalamus. Collateral branches of these axons separate from the tract and terminate in several nuclei, including the facial nucleus, motor nucleus of the trigeminal nerve, and various nuclei of the brainstem reticular formation.

9. Axons arising from cells of the principal nucleus of the trigeminal nerve project to the ventral posteromedial (VPM) nucleus of the thalamus via two pathways. Some cells give rise to axons that cross the midline and join the ventral trigeminothalamic tract, while others ascend on the ipsilateral side, forming the dorsal trigeminothalamic tract. Both pathways terminate in the VPM nucleus of the thalamus.

10. The principal trigeminal nucleus is different from the spinal trigeminal nucleus not only in that it receives nerve impulses from predominantly non-nociceptive receptors, but it also receives information from predominantly the perioral and intraoral distribution of the trigeminal nerve.

11. Nerve cell bodies in the VPM nucleus of the thalamus are the origin of projections to the lateral part of the postcentral gyrus. Thalamocortical projections arising from VPM lie in the posterior limb of the internal capsule and terminate somatotopically in the postcentral gyrus (primary sensory cortex) with the lower part of the face projected upon the more inferior (suprasylvian) part of the gyrus and upper part of the face projected more superiorly.

12. The motor division of the trigeminal nerve originates from the motor nucleus of the trigeminal nerve (masticator nucleus) located in the rostral pons. The axons of these lower motor neurons pass through the trigeminal ganglion and distribute to the muscles of mastication (masseter, temporalis, medial pterygoid, and lateral pterygoid) by way of branches of the mandibular nerve. The trigeminal nerve, the nerve of the first branchial arch, also provides motor innervation to other muscles derived from the first branchial arch, namely the tensor tympani, tensor veli palatini, anterior belly of the digastric, and mylohyoid.

13. The lower motor neurons of the motor nucleus of the trigeminal nerve receive synaptic input from the cerebral cortex and from several nuclei of the brainstem. Cortical input to the motor nucleus of the trigeminal nerve originates from cells in the lateral part of the precentral gyrus. The axons of these cells descend through the corona radiata and pass through the genu of the internal capsule and medial part of the cerebral peduncle. In the pons, they distribute bilaterally to the lower

motor neurons of the masticator nucleus. The nucleus also receives synaptic input from the mesencephalic nucleus of the trigeminal nerve as indicated above and from cells in the spinal trigeminal nucleus. This latter projection may be part of a mechanism for coordinating chewing and related jaw movements in response to tactile stimuli in the mouth.

14. Three important reflexes involving the trigeminal nerve are the corneal reflex, the masseter reflex, and the sneeze reflex. Branches of the trigeminal nerve serve as the afferent limb of each of these reflexes.

15. The ophthalmic branch of the trigeminal nerve functions as the afferent limb of the corneal reflex. Central processes of trigeminal ganglion cells descend in the spinal trigeminal tract to the level of the pontomedullary junction, where they synapse in the spinal trigeminal nucleus. Interneurons connect the spinal trigeminal nucleus with the facial nucleus on both sides of the brainstem. The facial nerve innervating the orbicularis oculi serves as the efferent limb of the corneal reflex. This reflex is characterized by bilateral closure of the palpebral fissures in response to tactile stimulation of the cornea (Figure 5-17).

16. The mandibular branch of the trigeminal nerve functions as the afferent limb of the masseter reflex. Central processes of cells in the mesencephalic nucleus project to and terminate on the alpha motor nucleus of the trigeminal motor nucleus. Interneurons interconnect the motor nuclei of the two sides. The mandibular nerve innervating the masseter muscle serves as the efferent limb of the masseter reflex. This reflex is characterized by closure of the jaw in response to sudden elongation (stretch) of the muscles of mastication (Figure 5-18).

17. The ophthalmic branch of the trigeminal nerve functions as the afferent limb of the sneeze reflex. Central processes of trigeminal ganglion cells descend in the spinal trigeminal tract to the level of the medulla oblongata, where they synapse in the spinal trigeminal nucleus and in nuclei of the reticular formation. Interneurons connect the spinal trigeminal nucleus with the nucleus ambiguus and motor neurons in the ventral horn of the spinal cord, specifically those that innervate the intercostal muscles and the diaphragm. The efferent limb of the sneeze reflex is made up of peripheral nerves that contribute the forceful exhalation. This reflex is characterized by forceful expulsion of air from the lungs in response to tactile stimulation of the mucosa of the nasal cavity.

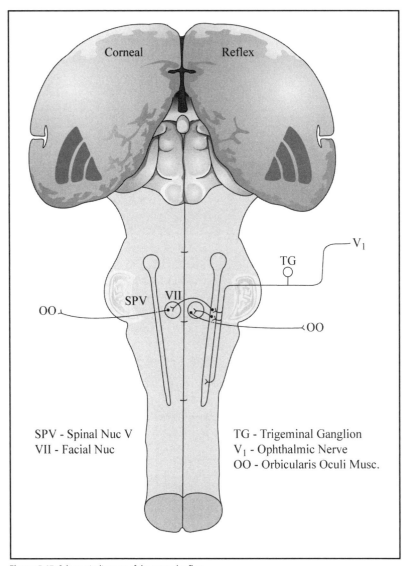

Figure 5-17: Schematic diagram of the corneal reflex.

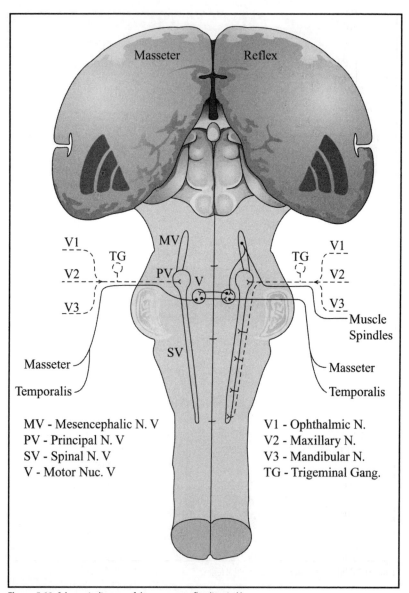

Figure 5-18: Schematic diagram of the masseter reflex (jaw jerk).

FACIAL NERVE

Key Points

1. The main functions of the facial nerve are to provide motor innervation to the muscles of facial expression and the lacrimal gland and to mediate taste from the anterior two-thirds of the tongue. It also serves as the efferent limb of the corneal and lacrimation reflexes.

2. The facial nerve emerges from the brainstem at the pontomedullary junction, immediately medial to the attachment of the vestibular division of the vestibulocochlear nerve. The axons of this mixed cranial nerve are organized to form two grossly distinct bundles—a physically larger collection of axons generally referred to as the *facial nerve proper* and a smaller bundle of axons known as the *nervus intermedius*. The facial nerve proper is formed by the axons of lower motor neurons that innervate striated muscles derived from the second branchial arch (ie, muscles of facial expression). The smaller nervus intermedius is composed of afferent axons, largely from taste buds on the anterior two-thirds of the tongue and autonomic axons involved in the innervation of the lacrimal gland and the sublingual and submandibular salivary glands (Figure 5-19).

3. The axons that innervate striated muscles arise from alpha motor neurons located in the caudal part of the pons in the facial nucleus. Within the brainstem, these axons initially course dorsomedially from the facial nucleus toward the abducens nucleus over which they pass, forming an elevation in the floor of the fourth ventricle known as the *facial colliculus*. The axons then course ventrolaterally through the lateral part of the pontine reticular formation to emerge from the brainstem in association with the nervus intermedius and vestibular nerve. The term *internal genu of the facial nerve* is used to describe these axons as they pass over the abducens nucleus, between the nucleus and the ependymal lining of the floor of the fourth ventricle. Upon exiting the brainstem, the axons pass through the internal auditory meatus together with the nervus intermedius and both divisions of the vestibulocochlear nerve. A short distance within the petrous part of the temporal bone, the axons pass through the geniculate ganglion to course posteriorly within the bone, medial to the middle ear, and then inferiorly to leave the skull by way of the stylomastoid foramen. Outside the skull, these axons invade the parotid gland where they divide into the five terminal branches of the facial nerve: *temporal, zygomatic, buccal, marginal mandibular,*

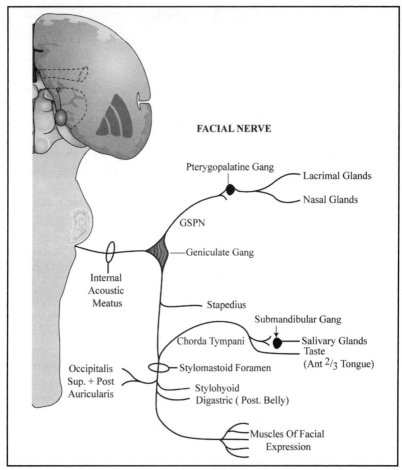

Figure 5-19: Schematic diagram of peripheral nervous system structures associated with the facial nerve. GSPN=Greater superficial petrosal nerve.

and *cervical*. A branch (nerve to the stapedius) arises from the facial nerve within the temporal bone, distal to the geniculate ganglion. The action of the stapedius muscle is to restrict movement of the stapes, specifically, movement of its footplate in the oval window. The action of the stapedius muscle will therefore dampen or reduce stimulus delivered to the organ of Corti.

4. The afferent axons in the facial nerve originate largely from chemoreceptors located in taste buds distributed on the anterior two-thirds of the tongue. These visceral afferent axons initially travel

with the lingual branch of the trigeminal nerve in the oral cavity, but later peel off and form part of the chorda tympani near the base of the skull. The chorda tympani passes through the middle ear medial to the tympanic membrane and joins the facial nerve within the temporal bone slightly above the stylomastoid foramen. The cell bodies of these visceral afferent axons are located in the geniculate ganglion. The central processes of these cells form part of the nervus intermedius and enter the brainstem as previously described. Within the brainstem, these axons join with other visceral afferent fibers subserving taste, forming the rostral part of the solitary tract. The axons of the solitary tract terminate in the rostral part of the solitary nucleus, often referred to as the *gustatory nucleus.*

5. The solitary nucleus is a visceral association nucleus, and as such receives synaptic input from visceral afferent fibers, both special (taste) and general (touch and thermal). (*Note*: Visceral afferent axons entering the brainstem by way of other cranial nerves will also synapse in the solitary nucleus.)

6. The visceral association cells of the solitary nucleus, including the gustatory nucleus, give rise to axons that terminate in nuclei of the thalamus and hypothalamus, as well as nearby nuclei in the brainstem. Projections to the thalamus terminate largely in the medial most part of the ventral posteromedial nucleus, which in turn projects axons via the posterior limb of the internal capsule to the opercular part of the postcentral gyrus (Brodmann area 43). This area of the parietal cortex is functionally considered to be primary gustatory cortex. Projections to the hypothalamus are thought to be important in regulating hypothalamic responses to gustatory stimuli. Projections from the solitary nucleus to other brainstem nuclei (dorsal motor nucleus of X, superior and inferior salivatory nuclei, nucleus ambiguus, hypoglossal nucleus, facial nucleus, masticator nucleus) help to regulate other functions related to gustatory stimulation such as gut motility, salivation, pharyngeal muscle contraction, tongue movement, buccinator muscle contraction, and mandibular movements, all of which are important in food intake, mastication, swallowing, and digestion (Figure 5-20).

7. The autonomic efferent axons of the facial nerve originate in the caudal pons from cells that form the superior salivatory nucleus. Functionally, the cells of the superior salivatory nucleus are defined as preganglionic parasympathetic cells. The axons of these cells exit the brainstem and pass through the internal auditory meatus as part of the nervus intermedius. Upon reaching the geniculate ganglion, some of the preganglionic axons separate and course anteromedially

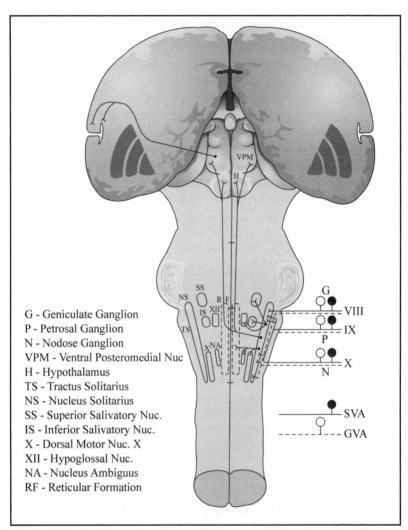

G - Geniculate Ganglion
P - Petrosal Ganglion
N - Nodose Ganglion
VPM - Ventral Posteromedial Nuc
H - Hypothalamus
TS - Tractus Solitarius
NS - Nucleus Solitarius
SS - Superior Salivatory Nuc.
IS - Inferior Salivatory Nuc.
X - Dorsal Motor Nuc. X
XII - Hypoglossal Nuc.
NA - Nucleus Ambiguus
RF - Reticular Formation

Figure 5-20: Schematic diagram of the afferent and efferent connections of the solitary nucleus. SVA=special visceral afferent cell, GVA=general visceral afferent cell.

in the floor of the middle cranial fossa as the greater petrosal nerve, while others continue through the temporal bone together with the axons of the facial nerve proper. The greater petrosal nerve passes into the pterygoid (vidian) canal and emerges in the pterygopalatine fossa, where the fibers terminate by making synaptic contact with postganglionic parasympathetic nerve cell bodies of the pterygopalatine ganglion. The axons of these latter cells enter the orbit by way of the inferior orbital fissure as part of the maxillary nerve. Within the orbit, these axons separate from the zygomatic branch of the maxillary nerve to join the lacrimal branch of the ophthalmic nerve and by way of this nerve, are distributed to the lacrimal gland. The remaining preganglionic parasympathetic fibers course with the facial nerve within the temporal bone to a point slightly superior to the stylomastoid foramen. At this point, the axons separate from the facial nerve and join the chorda tympani, which passes through the middle ear cavity to emerge from the base of the skull through a small opening located just medial to the spine of the sphenoid bone. The axons then join the lingual branch of the mandibular nerve to enter the oral cavity, where they terminate on postganglionic parasympathetic cell bodies of the submandibular ganglion. The axons of these latter cells then project to the submandibular and sublingual glands (Figure 5-21).

8. The muscles of facial expression receive motor innervation by way of alpha motor neurons (lower motor neurons) located in the ipsilateral facial nucleus. The facial nucleus receives synaptic input from nerve cell bodies located in the cerebral cortex (cortical upper motor neurons) and from several nuclei located within the brainstem (brainstem upper motor neurons). Cortical upper motor neurons are located in the precentral gyrus, where they are somatotopically organized with neurons subserving upper facial muscles located superior to those influencing muscles of the lower part of the face. The axons of these cells descend through the corona radiata, genu of the internal capsule, medial portion of the cerebral peduncle, and medial part of the longitudinal pontine bundles. Near the level of the caudal pons, some of these corticonuclear axons decussate to terminate on the contralateral side. The facial nucleus is innervated such that those lower motor neurons that innervate the muscles of the lower half of the face (ie, zygomaticus major and orbicularis oris) receive synaptic input from the cortical cells on the contralateral side only while lower motor neurons that innervate muscles of the upper half of the face (ie, frontalis and orbicularis oculi) receive synaptic input from cortical cells on both sides. The facial nuclei are also influenced, probably indirectly, by cortical areas of the limbic system. The evidence for this later innervation pattern is derived from patients who are unable to contract their facial musculature on a voluntary basis but are able to do so in response to some emotionally charged event or experience (Figure 5-22).

9. The facial nucleus also receives synaptic input from several brainstem nuclei, including the spinal trigeminal nucleus, superior olivary

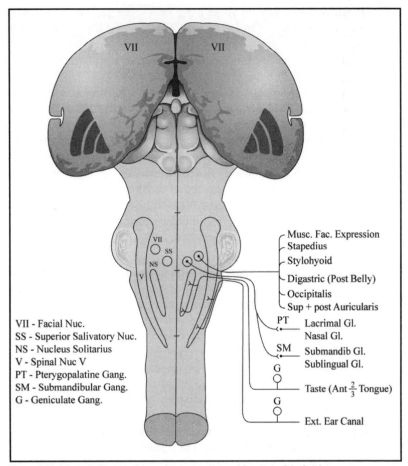

Figure 5-21: Schematic diagram of the nuclear connections and functions of the facial nerve.

nuclei, and the solitary nucleus. Connections between these nuclei and the facial nucleus mediate a number of reflex responses stimulated by tactile, auditory, and gustatory stimuli. Among these reflexes are the lacrimal reflex, salivation reflex, corneal reflex, the startle response, and several developmental (or pathological) reflexes such as the snout reflex and the suck and rooting reflexes (Figures 5-23 and 5-24).

10. Signs and symptoms associated with lesions that interrupt transmission in the facial nerve depend on the location of the lesion within the cranial vault, skull, or outside the skull. As a result, the location

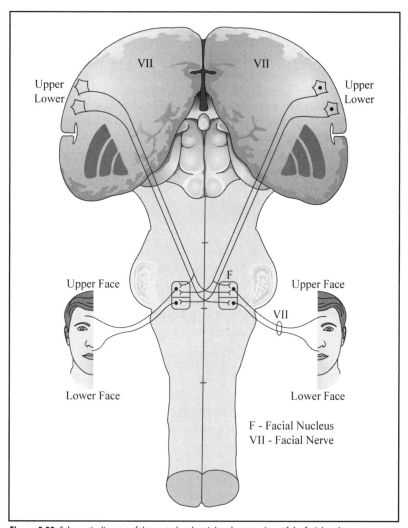

Upper
Lower

VII

VII

Upper
Lower

Upper Face

F

Upper Face

VII

Lower Face

Lower Face

F - Facial Nucleus
VII - Facial Nerve

Figure 5-22: Schematic diagram of the central and peripheral connections of the facial nucleus.

of lesions affecting the facial nerve can be easily determined by a careful and thorough assessment of facial nerve function. With regard to lesions that damage the facial nucleus or its axons anywhere along their course (lower motor neuron lesions), the resulting facial paresis or paralysis will always be ipsilateral to the lesion. Facial paralysis or paresis of idiopathic origin (unknown etiology) is referred to as *Bell's*

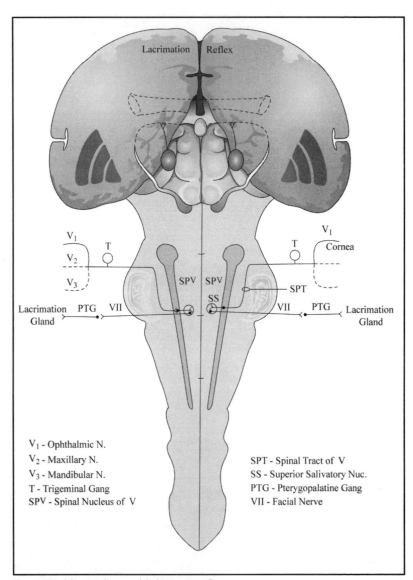

Figure 5-23: Schematic diagram of the lacrimation reflex.

palsy. Lesions that damage the face region of the precentral gyrus (primary motor cortex) or the axons of corticonuclear projections to the facial nucleus on one side (upper motor neuron lesions) result in facial paralysis or paresis involving the lower half of the face on the contralateral side only (muscle function in the upper half of the face

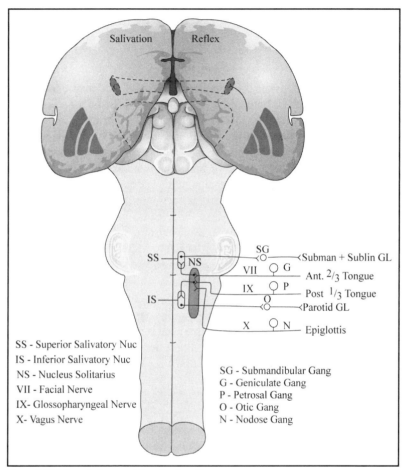

Figure 5-24: Schematic diagram of the salivation reflex.

remains functionally intact bilaterally). Patients with facial paralysis resulting from lower motor neuron involvement are typically unable to fully close the eye on the involved side (ie, contract the orbicularis oculi sufficiently to approximate the upper and lower lids). If you ask such a patient to forcefully close the lids, and carefully observe the eye on the involved side, you will note that the eye supraducts, revealing the sclera below the cornea. Supraduction of the eye associated with attempts at forceful closure of the lids is known as *Bell's phenomenon* (not to be confused with Bell's palsy), and represents a normal response that probably evolved to help further protect the light transmitting structures of the eye from trauma.

AUDITORY SYSTEM

Key Points

1. Sound waves passing through the external auditory canal cause movement of the tympanic membrane, which in turn causes movement of the malleus, incus, and stapes within the middle ear cavity, which in turn produces compression and rarefaction waves in the perilymph fluid in the scala vestibuli and scala tympani, which in turn causes movement of the basilar membrane, which in turn induces bending of the stereocilia of the auditory receptor cells, which in turn depolarizes or hyperpolarizes these cells as a result of the opening and closing of mechanically gated ion channels located in the stereocilia cell membrane. Depolarization of an auditory receptor cell results in the transmission of nerve impulses (action potentials) toward the CNS by way of the cochlear nerve (cochlear division of the vestibulocochlear nerve).

2. Auditory receptor cells (inner and outer hair cells) rest on the basilar membrane surrounded by endolymph in the scala media (cochlear duct). The apical end of the receptor cell is characterized by stereocilia that make physical contact with the tectorial membrane, also located within the cochlear duct. Auditory receptor cells are depolarized or hyperpolarized as a result of bending of the stereocilia secondary to movement of the basilar membrane.

3. The basilar membrane in humans is approximately 33 mm in length when uncoiled. It is wider at its apex than at its base. As a consequence, auditory receptor cells located near the base are preferentially activated by higher frequency tones, while hair cells near the apex (*helicotrema*) preferentially respond to low frequency tones. Thus, auditory receptor cells are said to be tonotopically organized on the basilar membrane, with high frequency tones represented near the base of the organ of Corti and low tones represented nearer the apex.

4. Depolarization of auditory receptor cells results in the transmission of nerve impulses toward the CNS by way of the *cochlear nerve* (cochlear division of the vestibulocochlear nerve). The cell bodies of these neural crest-derived afferent cells are bipolar in form and comprise the spiral ganglion, located within the modiolus of the cochlea. The peripheral processes are short and make synaptic contact with the auditory receptor cells, while the central processes are comparatively long and form the cochlear nerve. Approximately 95% of the axons of the cochlear nerve are afferent in function. Approximately

95% of these transmit nerve impulses from the inner hair cells. The remaining afferent fibers transmit from the outer hair cells.

5. The central processes of spiral ganglion cells pass through the internal auditory meatus together with the vestibular nerve and the facial nerve, including its smaller component, the nervus intermedius, to enter the middle cranial fossa. The axons of the cochlear nerve enter the brainstem at the level of the rostral medulla oblongata and terminate by making synaptic contact with cells in the dorsal and ventral cochlear nuclei. These nuclei are located on the dorsolateral and lateral surface, respectively, of the inferior cerebellar peduncle, immediately caudal to the cerebellum. Like the organ of Corti, the dorsal and ventral cochlear nuclei are tonotopically organized. Cells responsive to high frequency tones are located dorsomedial within each nucleus, with those responsive to low frequency tones being located in a more ventrolateral location. Lesions involving the cochlear nerve or cochlear nuclei result in hearing impairments on the ipsilateral side (Figure 5-25).

6. Projections from the cochlear nuclei terminate in several nuclei of the brainstem and thalamus, including the nucleus of the inferior colliculus and the medial geniculate nucleus. Axons of the smaller dorsal cochlear nucleus cross the midline in the dorsal part of the pontine tegmentum by way of a small bundle known as the *dorsal acoustic stria*. After crossing the midline, these fibers ascend to the level of the midbrain as part of the lateral lemniscus. Most of the fibers of the lateral lemniscus terminate in the nucleus of the inferior colliculus. Axons of the larger ventral cochlear nucleus cross the midline in the intermediate and ventral part of the pontine tegmentum, where they form the intermediate and ventral acoustic stria, respectively. The ventral acoustic stria is also known as the *trapezoid body*. Axons originating in the ventral cochlear nuclei terminate mainly in the contralateral nucleus of the inferior colliculus and bilaterally in the superior olivary nuclei. The superior olivary nucleus is, in turn, the origin of both uncrossed, but predominantly crossed projections that course by way of the lateral lemniscus to the nucleus of the inferior colliculus. The functional significance of this predominantly contralateral distribution of axons from the cochlear and superior olivary nuclei is that most (approximately 70%) of the auditory nerve impulses that leave the cochlear nuclei influence higher brain centers on the contralateral side. Clinically, this results in the observation that lesions involving the lateral lemniscus or medial geniculate nucleus will result in bilateral hearing impairment (*hypacusis*) with a greater hearing loss in the contralateral ear.

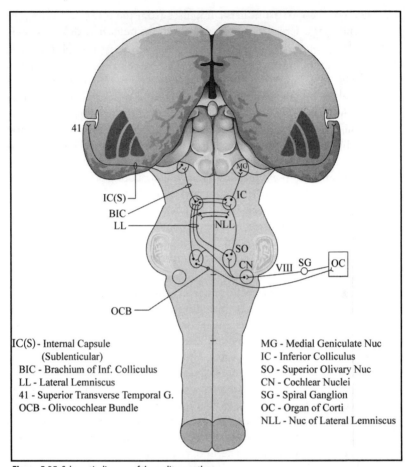

Figure 5-25: Schematic diagram of the auditory pathway.

7. The lateral lemniscus lies in the lateral part of the pontine tegmentum. Most of the axons terminate in the ipsilateral inferior colliculus, with a few extending further rostrally to end in the medial geniculate nucleus. Cells of the nucleus of the inferior colliculus give rise to two short pathways; one, the brachium of the inferior colliculus, extends rostrally to terminate in the medial geniculate and the other, the commissure of the inferior colliculus, crosses the midline to terminate in the inferior colliculus of the opposite side. The nucleus of the inferior colliculus appears to play a role in reflex eye and head movements that occur in response to auditory stimuli.

8. The nerve cells that form the medial geniculate nucleus, like those of the cochlear nuclei, are tonotopically organized with those that respond to high frequency tones located in the dorsomedial part of the nucleus and those responding to low frequency tones distributed in the ventrolateral part of the nucleus.

9. The cells of the medial geniculate nucleus are the origin of axons that terminate on the ipsilateral side in the superior transverse temporal gyrus (*Heschl's convolution*) of the temporal lobe. These thalamo-cortical (geniculocortical) projections reach the superior transverse temporal gyrus by passing through a region of the subcortical white matter frequently referred to as the *sublenticular part of the internal capsule* (more properly, the sublenticular part of the posterior limb of the internal capsule). Like other parts of the auditory system, the superior transverse temporal gyrus is tonotopically organized with high frequency tones exciting cells located in the posteromedial part of the gyrus and low frequency tones activating cells in the anterolateral part of the gyrus.

10. The main function of the cells in Heschl's convolution is auditory perception. The superior transverse temporal gyrus is functionally referred to as *primary auditory cortex* and represents Brodmann area 41. The blood supply to the primary auditory cortex is by way of cortical branches (M4) of the middle cerebral artery.

11. Sound recognition and interpretation are functions of adjacent cortical areas of the temporal lobe. These areas, including the planum temporale, are referred to as *auditory association areas* and correspond to Brodmann areas 42 and 22 of the temporal lobe. The arterial blood supply to the auditory association cortex is also by way of branches of the middle cerebral artery.

12. Lesions that damage the tympanic membrane or impair the movements of the ossicles of the middle ear result in hearing deficits generally referred to as *conduction deficits*. Lesions that damage the auditory receptor cells, the spiral ganglion cells or their axons, or the cochlear nuclei result in hearing abnormalities that are referred to as *sensorineural deficits*. Both types of deficits will affect hearing in the ipsilateral ear. The Rinne and Weber tests can be used to differentiate between conduction and sensorineural type hearing impairments.

13. Lesions that damage the primary auditory cortex or disrupt the projections from the medial geniculate nucleus to the primary auditory cortex can also impair hearing. The impairment is typically *hypacusis* (increased threshold to sound perception) in the contralateral ear together with a reduced ability to precisely localize sounds originating on the contralateral side.

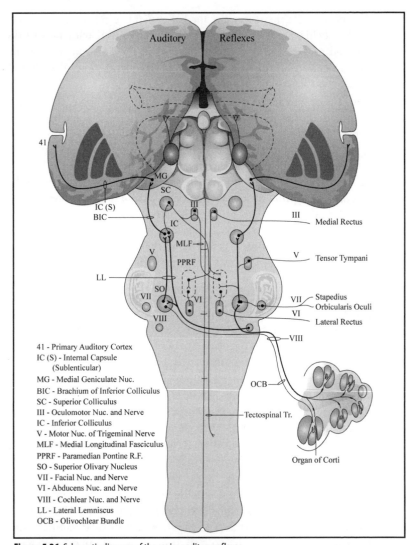

Auditory   Reflexes

41

MG
SC
IC (S)
BIC   III
III   ——— Medial Rectus
IC
MLF
V   V
PPRF   ——— Tensor Tympani
LL
SO
VII   VII — Stapedius
VI   Orbicularis Oculi
VIII   VI
                       ——— Lateral Rectus
                       VIII

41 - Primary Auditory Cortex
IC (S) - Internal Capsule
        (Sublenticular)
MG - Medial Geniculate Nuc.   OCB
BIC - Brachium of Inferior Colliculus
SC - Superior Colliculus
III - Oculomotor Nuc. and Nerve
IC - Inferior Colliculus   Tectospinal Tr.
V - Motor Nuc. of Trigeminal Nerve
MLF - Medial Longitudinal Fasciculus
PPRF - Paramedian Pontine R.F.
SO - Superior Olivary Nucleus
VII - Facial Nuc. and Nerve   Organ of Corti
VI - Abducens Nuc. and Nerve
VIII - Cochlear Nuc. and Nerve
LL - Lateral Lemniscus
OCB - Olivochlear Bundle

Figure 5-26: Schematic diagram of the major auditory reflexes.

14. Several auditory reflexes are known that serve to protect the auditory structures from mechanical damage resulting from loud noises. These reflexes involve contraction of the tensor tympani and stapedius muscles to dampen movement of the tympanic membrane and stapes, respectively. Contraction of these muscles restricts movement of the ossicles and thereby reduces perilymph wave production in the scala vestibuli and scala tympani (Figure 5-26).

15. Sound also excites a small population of efferent cells in the superior olivary nucleus. These cells are the origin of axons that exit the brainstem as part of the cochlear nerve and terminate on outer hair cells within the organ of Corti, predominantly on the contralateral side. These efferent axons, which constitute approximately 5% of the cochlear nerve, are known as the *olivocochlear bundles*. They affect hearing by influencing the excitability of the outer hair cells.

VESTIBULAR SYSTEM

Key Points

1. The major functions of the vestibular system are to help maintain visual fixation during locomotion and to support the head and body against the force of gravity.

2. The peripheral vestibular apparatus consists of five distinct receptor structures located within the petrous part of the temporal bone on each side. These receptor structures include the crista ampullaris located in each of the three semicircular canals, and the macula lutea located in the utricle and saccule. The receptors in the semicircular canals are responsive to rotational movements of the head (angular acceleration and deceleration) and only respond to changes in the velocity of head rotation. (They are silent when the head is at rest or when the head is rotating at a constant velocity.) The receptors in the utricle and saccule (otolithic organs) are responsive to linear movements of the head as well as static head position. Some of the cells in the utricle and saccule are responsive to the pull of gravity acting on the head. Movement of the head in any plane or about any axis produces excitation (depolarization) of specific receptor cells on one side of the head and inhibition (hyperpolarization) of specific receptor cells on the other side of the head.

3. The cell bodies of the vestibular nerve form the vestibular (Scarpa's) ganglion. The short peripheral processes of these bipolar afferent cells extend to make synaptic contact with the hair cell located in the ampulla of the semicircular canal or the macula of the saccule or utricle. The central processes pass through the internal auditory meatus and enter the brainstem at the level of the cerebello-medullary junction. Within the brainstem, the axons course dorsomedially toward the floor of the fourth ventricle, passing between the inferior cerebellar peduncle and the spinal trigeminal tract. Vestibular afferent axons terminate on the ipsilateral side, with most ending in the vestibular nuclei and a few passing directly into the cerebellum by way of the juxtarestiform body.

4. The vestibular nuclear complex is composed of four nuclei that lie in the lateral part of the floor of the fourth ventricle. The nuclear complex extends from the level of the mid-pons rostrally to mid-medullary levels caudally. These nuclei (superior, medial, lateral, and inferior) are the origin of axons that project to 1) gaze centers of the pons and midbrain; 2) spinal lower motor neurons that innervate axial extensor muscles and appendicular extensor muscles of the lower and upper limbs; 3) nuclei of the diencephalon including the thalamus and hypothalamus; 4) nuclei within the brainstem associated with eating, swallowing and GI motility; 5) brainstem reticular formation cells that influence preganglionic cells of the autonomic nervous system; and 6) the cerebellum (Figure 5-27).

5. Cells in the rostral part of the vestibular nuclear complex receive synaptic input predominantly from the semicircular canals and project axons by way of the *medial longitudinal fasciculus* (MLF) to caudal brainstem gaze centers, including the *nucleus prepositus* and *paramedian pontine reticular formation* (PPRF) and rostral brainstem gaze centers including the *rostral interstitial nucleus of the medial longitudinal fasciculus* (riMLF) and the *interstitial nucleus of Cajal* (INC). The gaze centers in turn, project axons by way of the MLF to the extraocular nuclei (oculomotor, trochlear, and abducens) and to cervical spinal cord levels, where they influence lower motor neurons that innervate neck muscles. This system of projections mediates automatic (reflex) eye movements in response to changes in head position generally referred to as the *vestibulo-ocular reflex*.

6. Cells in the caudal part of the vestibular nuclear complex receive synaptic input predominantly from the maculae of the saccule and utricle and project axons by way of the vestibulospinal tracts to influence spinal lower motor neurons (alpha and gamma) that innervate axial extensor muscles and extensor muscles of the lower and upper limbs. Lower motor neurons that innervate axial (predominantly cervical) extensor muscles are influenced by axons of the ventral vestibulospinal tract located in the ventral funiculus of the spinal cord. These axons arise chiefly from the inferior vestibular nucleus. Lower motor neurons that innervate appendicular extensor muscles are influenced by axons of the lateral vestibulospinal tract located in the ventrolateral fasciculus of the spinal cord. These axons arise exclusively from the lateral vestibular nucleus (*Deiter's nucleus*).

7. Cells of the vestibular nuclei project axons rostrally to the thalamus (VPM) and hypothalamus. Projections to the thalamus influence thalamocortical projections to the insula that likely play a role in the experience of nausea. Other projections, possibly through the VPM

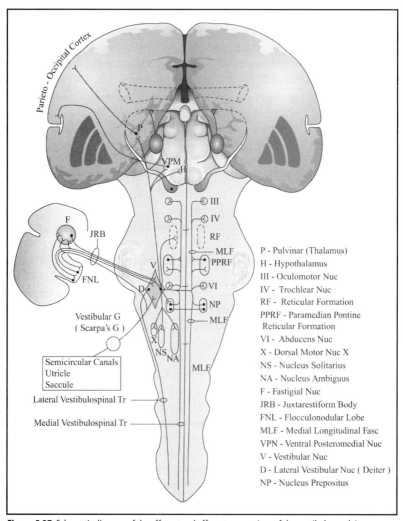

Figure 5-27: Schematic diagram of the afferent and efferent connections of the vestibular nuclei.

to the posterior part of the insular cortices, may be important in mediating the experience of vertigo. Projections to the hypothalamus likely participate in control of selected autonomic functions related to gastrointestinal function.

8. The vestibular nuclei project axons to the nucleus ambiguus, hypoglossal nucleus, and dorsal motor nucleus X, nuclei that influence

the muscles of the pharynx, tongue, esophagus, and stomach. The functional role of these projections in humans is limited. However, vestibular influences on these nuclei may be implicated in vomiting, a finding sometimes noted in individuals suffering from certain types of vestibular disorders.

9. The vestibular nuclei project axons to areas of the brainstem reticular formation known to influence autonomic nervous system activity. These areas are known to contain cells that give rise to descending pathways (reticulospinal pathways) that synapse on preganglionic sympathetic cells of the intermediolateral nucleus and preganglionic parasympathetic cells of the sacral parasympathetic nucleus. These descending pathways may be implicated in such findings as facial pallor, sweating, and other autonomic signs and symptoms sometimes seen in individuals with vestibular system dysfunction.

10. All of the vestibular nuclei give rise to axons that project to the ipsilateral cerebellum by way of the juxtarestiform body, a small phylogenetically old fiber tract located along the medial edge of the inferior cerebellar peduncle. Projections to the cerebellum terminate predominantly in the flocculonodular lobe, vermis, and fastigial nucleus, parts of the cerebellum that in turn give rise to projections that return to the vestibular nuclei by way of the juxtarestiform body. The role of the cerebellum seems to be to help sequence in **time**, the output of the vestibular nuclei to its various forebrain, brainstem, and spinal targets.

11. Signs and symptoms suggestive of vestibular system dysfunction are most commonly the result of an imbalance in the neural input to the vestibular nuclei from the two sides. Most commonly, vestibular signs and symptoms are associated with injuries or disease processes affecting the vestibular receptors or the vestibular nerve.

BULBAR CRANIAL NERVES

Key Points

1. Cranial Nerves III through XII are the segmental nerves of the brainstem. Unlike spinal nerves, which are classified as "mixed" nerves, cranial nerves are functionally classified as purely sensory, purely motor, or mixed.

2. The term *bulbar cranial nerves* refers to the cranial nerves associated with the medulla oblongata (the "bulb"). These include the glossopharyngeal (IX), vagus (X), spinal accessory (XI), and

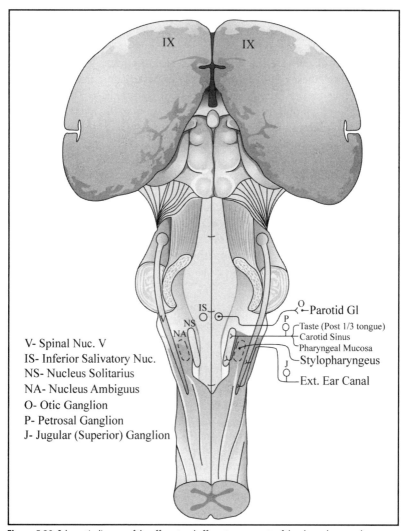

Figure 5-28: Schematic diagram of the afferent and efferent components of the glossopharyngeal nerve.

hypoglossal (XII). Cranial nerves IX and X are mixed and cranial nerves XI and XII are classified as purely motor.

3. The glossopharyngeal nerve (CN IX) is a mixed nerve with both afferent and efferent functions (Figure 5-28). *Afferent* cell bodies form two ganglia: a small superior (jugular) ganglion, typically located

within the jugular foramen and a slightly larger inferior (petrosal) ganglion positioned immediately below the jugular foramen. Axons of cells in the superior ganglion innervate a small area of skin in the region of the external auditory canal and auricle. The central processes of these cells terminate in the spinal trigeminal nucleus. Axons of cells in the inferior ganglion (petrosal ganglion) innervate taste buds on the posterior one-third of the tongue, the mucosal lining of the oropharynx in the region of the soft palate and tonsillar fossa, and the baroreceptors of the carotid sinus. The central processes of these axons terminate in the nucleus solitarius, including its rostral extent, sometimes referred to as the *gustatory nucleus*. *Efferent* axons arise from cells in the nucleus ambiguus and the inferior salivatory nucleus. Those that originate in the nucleus ambiguus innervate the stylopharyngeus muscle. Those that originate in the inferior salivatory nucleus (preganglionic parasympathetic cells) terminate in the otic ganglion on postganglionic parasympathetic cells that innervate the parotid gland. The glossopharyngeal nerve serves as the afferent limb of the pharyngeal (gag) reflex.

4. The vagus nerve (CN X) is a mixed nerve with both afferent and efferent functions (Figure 5-29). Similar to the glossopharyngeal nerve, afferent cell bodies of the vagus nerve form two ganglia: a small superior (jugular) ganglion, typically located within the jugular foramen and a slightly larger inferior (nodose) ganglion positioned immediately below the jugular foramen. Axons of cells in the superior ganglion innervate a small area of skin in the region of the external auditory canal and auricle. The central processes of these cells terminate in the spinal trigeminal nucleus. Axons of cells in the inferior ganglion (nodose ganglion) innervate taste buds on the epiglottis and chemoreceptors of the carotid body. The majority of the visceral afferent fibers of the vagus nerve innervate the mucosal lining of the digestive tract from the esophagus to approximately the level of the left colic (splenic) flexure of the large intestine. These fibers also provide sensory innervation to the visceral pleura, visceral pericardium, and the organs of the abdominal cavity. Embryologically, receptors associated with visceral afferent fibers are located in tissues derived from primitive endoderm and splanchnic mesoderm. The central processes of these visceral afferent fibers terminate in the nucleus solitarius, including its rostral extent, the *gustatory nucleus*. Efferent axons of the vagus nerve arise from cells in the nucleus ambiguus and dorsal motor nucleus (of the vagus nerve). Cells of the nucleus ambiguus are the origin of axons that innervate branchial arch-derived, striated muscles of the pharynx (pharyngeal constrictors), the levator veli

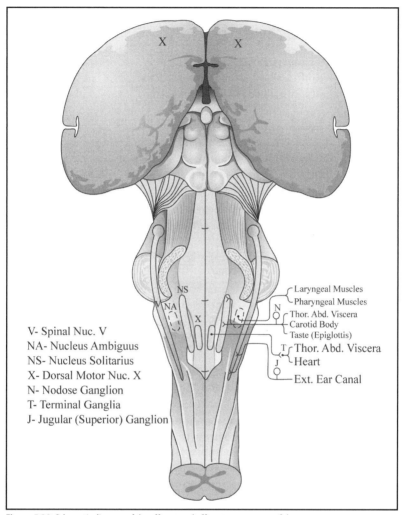

Figure 5-29: Schematic diagram of the afferent and efferent components of the vagus nerve.

palatini, and the muscles of the larynx. Cortical upper motor neurons that influence the nucleus ambiguus are located both ipsilateral and contralateral to the nucleus. Cells of the dorsal motor nucleus are preganglionic parasympathetic cells that innervate postganglionic parasympathetic cells in the *terminal ganglia*, including those that are part of the pulmonary and cardiac plexuses. Parasympathetic innervation to the GI tract mediated by the vagus nerve extends approximately to the level of the left colic (splenic) flexure of the large colon. Important functions of the vagus nerve include monitoring arterial blood gasses by way of chemoreceptors in the carotid body; innervation of the muscles of the larynx involved in speaking and breathing; innervation of the pharyngeal constrictors involved in swallowing; innervation of gastric and intestinal glands involved in digestion and absorption of materials from the GI tract; innervation of esophageal, gastric, and intestinal smooth muscle involved in peristaltic activity of the GI tract; innervation of cardiac muscle (slows heart rate); and innervation of tracheo-bronchial and esophageal mucosa in relation to the protective cough and gag reflexes, respectively (Figure 5-30).

5. The spinal accessory nerve (CN XI) is a motor nerve. The cell bodies of the accessory nerve are located in the accessory nucleus located in the intermediate gray of the spinal cord at the C1 – C4 cord levels. The axons of these cells exit the spinal cord as a separate lateral root and collect into a bundle that ascends within the spinal subarachnoid space to enter the skull through the foramen magnum. Within the posterior cranial fossa, the axons of the accessory nerve course laterally together with those of the vagus nerve toward the jugular foramen through which they both pass. The two nerves separate within or immediately outside the jugular foramen. The axons of the accessory nerve pass inferiorly to provide motor innervation to the trapezius and sternocleidomastoid. Cortical projections to the accessory nucleus originate predominantly in the ipsilateral hemisphere (Figure 5-31).

6. The hypoglossal nerve (CN XII) is a motor nerve. The cell bodies of the hypoglossal nerve are located in the hypoglossal nucleus located near the midline in the rostral part of the medulla oblongata. The axons of these cells pass ventrolaterally through the medulla to exit the brainstem at the preolivary sulcus. The axons exit the skull by passing through the hypoglossal canal to reach and innervate the intrinsic and extrinsic muscles of the tongue. Cortical upper motor neurons that influence the hypoglossal nucleus are located contralateral to the nucleus. The intrinsic muscles of the tongue form the bulk of the tongue and undergo atrophic changes when denervated as a result of lesions involving the hypoglossal nerve. The extrinsic muscles of the tongue (*genioglossus, hyoglossus, styloglossus,* and *palatoglossus*) operate to move the tongue as a unit. The genioglossus muscle is important in tongue protrusion and is the muscle most frequently tested in the routine neurological examination. The palatoglossus is the only extrinsic muscle of the tongue not innervated by the hypoglossal nerve (it is innervated by the vagus nerve). Cortical projections to

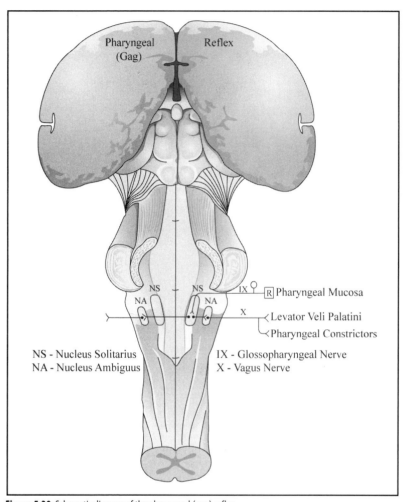

Figure 5-30: Schematic diagram of the pharyngeal (gag) reflex.

the hypoglossal nucleus originate in the contralateral hemisphere. Lesions involving the hypoglossal nerve are characterized by atrophy of the ipsilateral half of the tongue, *dysarthria* for lingual sounds, and difficulty with moving food within the mouth in relation to chewing and swallowing (*dysphagia*). The tongue deviates to the ipsilateral side when protruded (Figure 5-32).

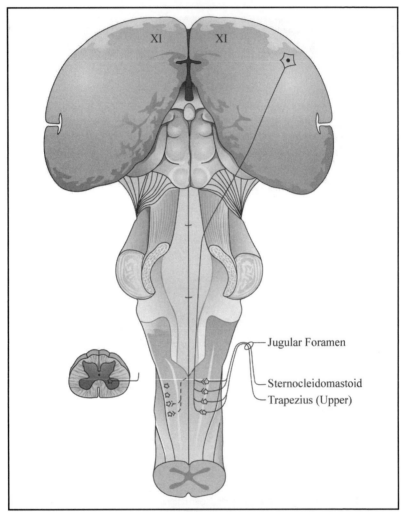

Figure 5-31: Schematic diagram of the upper and lower motor neuron components of the spinal accessory nerve.

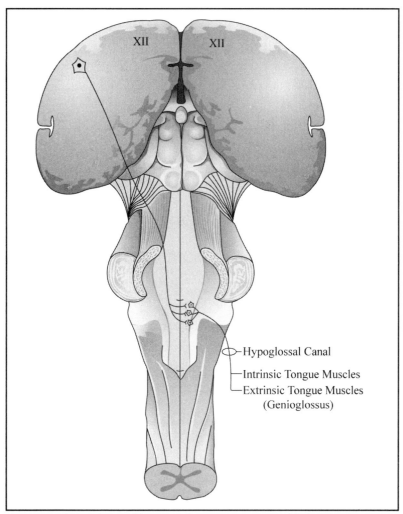

Figure 5-32: Schematic diagram of the upper and lower motor components of the hypoglossal nerve.

SECTION VI

Cortical Organization and Higher Brain Functions

Nolan M.
*Cram Session in Functional Neuroanatomy:
A Handbook for Students & Clinicians* (pp. 171-188)
© 2012 SLACK Incorporated

CEREBRAL CORTEX AND SUBCORTICAL WHITE MATTER

Key Points

1. The human *cerebral cortex* is a relatively thin layer of gray matter (neuronal cell bodies) located on the surface of the cerebral hemisphere. The cells of the cerebral cortex are bounded superficially and separated from the innermost layer of the pia matter (intima pia) by *glial foot processes*. Deep to the cerebral cortex is the *subcortical white matter*, a region composed of axons and their myelin sheaths.

2. The surface of the brain is not smooth but is rather thrown into folds referred to as *gyri*. Clefts or spaces between adjacent gyri are known as *fissures* or *sulci*. Fissures and/or sulci commonly serve as boundaries to delimit lobes of the brain or smaller regions within a particular lobe. More than half of the cortical surface is not visible when looking at the intact gross brain. Most of the cortical surface forms the walls and floor of the various sulci and fissures.

3. Sulci, fissures, and gyri are commonly designated by name. In addition, many regions of the cerebral cortex are also identified by number, the most common numbering system being one described by Brodmann. Although some gyri have a specific Brodmann number, there is not always direct correspondence between the name of a particular gyrus and a Brodmann number.

4. The human brain is commonly divided into four lobes: *frontal, parietal, occipital,* and *temporal.* (*Note*: Additional "lobes" have been described in the literature. Some authors have used the term *insular lobe* when referring collectively to the long and short gyri of the insula. Others have used the term *limbic lobe* when referring to the cortical areas functionally associated with the limbic system, namely the dentate gyrus, parahippocampal gyrus, isthmus of the hippocampal, cingulate gyrus, subcallosal gyrus, and paraterminal gyrus.)

5. In humans, approximately 41% of the cortical surface is part of the frontal lobe. The parietal and temporal lobes account for approximately 21% each, and the occipital lobe accounts for approximately 17% of the cortical surface.

6. Based on both functional and anatomical studies, it has become convenient to recognize three types of cortical areas: *primary cortex* (motor and sensory), *modality-specific association cortex,* and *integrative association cortex.* The primary sensory and motor cortices

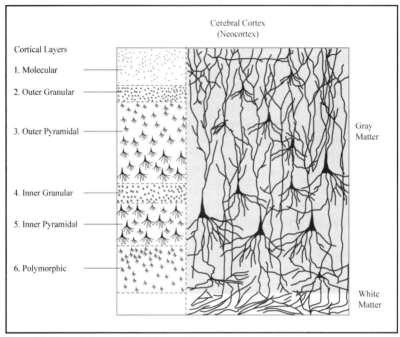

Cerebral Cortex
(Neocortex)

Cortical Layers

1. Molecular

2. Outer Granular

3. Outer Pyramidal

4. Inner Granular

5. Inner Pyramidal

6. Polymorphic

Gray
Matter

White
Matter

Figure 6-1: Schematic diagram of the six layers of the neocortex.

represent approximately 25% of the cortical structure. The remaining 75% is classified as association cortex, either modality-specific or integrative.

7. The human cerebral cortex is not histologically identical in all areas of the brain. The phylogenetically oldest cortical areas (archi and paleo cortex) consist of three layers of cells extending from the pia mater to the border with the subcortical white matter. In humans, these cortical areas account for approximately 10% of the total cortical surface and represent cortical areas associated with the limbic system. The remaining, approximately 90% of the cortical surface, (neo-cortex) presents a six-layered cortical structure. The six layers, from superficial to deep, are the *molecular, outer plexiform, outer pyramidal, inner plexiform, inner pyramidal,* and *polymorphic* (fusiform) (Figure 6-1).

8. The cerebral cortex is not of uniform thickness throughout the brain. Neocortical areas in particular range in thickness from 1.5 to 4.5 mm. These differences reflect the histological organization of the cortex in different regions of the hemisphere.

9. The subcortical white matter is a region of the telencephalon composed of myelinated axons. The lighter appearance of this part of the cerebral hemisphere (whiteness) is the consequence of the presence of myelin in the central nervous system (CNS). Myelin in the CNS is the tightly wrapped cell membranes of oligodendrocytes. The axons (fibers) forming the subcortical white are classified as projection, association, or commissural fibers based on the location of their cell bodies and synaptic endings (Figure 6-2).

10. Projection fibers interconnect specific cortical areas with specific nuclei outside the cerebral cortex. Projection fibers are classified as descending or ascending based on the direction of nerve impulse transmission. *Descending projection fibers* arise predominantly from cells in the inner pyramidal layer of the cerebral cortex and terminate in various nuclei of the forebrain, brainstem, and spinal cord. Those that terminate in the brainstem and spinal cord pass through the internal capsule. *Ascending projection fibers* arise predominantly from cells in particular nuclei of the dorsal thalamus, particular nuclei of the brainstem reticular formation, and particular nuclei of the forebrain, most notably the basal nucleus of Meynert. Thalamocortical projection fibers are found predominantly in the internal capsule. Reticulocortical projection fibers are found predominantly in the medial forebrain bundle.

11. Association fibers interconnect different cortical areas within the same hemisphere, thus forming intra-hemispheric connections. Short association fibers interconnect nearby areas. Longer association fibers interconnect cortical areas located further apart, such as areas of the occipital lobe with areas in the frontal lobe. These longer association fibers commonly form "bundles" called *fasciculi* located in specific regions of the subcortical white matter. Among the more commonly recognized intra-hemispheric association bundles are the superior longitudinal fasciculus, inferior longitudinal fasciculus, inferior fronto-occipital fasciculus, arcuate fasciculus, uncinate fasciculus, and the cingulum bundle (Figure 6-3).

12. Commissural fibers interconnect cortical areas in one hemisphere with cortical areas in the contralateral hemisphere. Commissural fibers form inter-hemispheric connections. Unlike projection fibers that either terminate on primary cortical cells (ascending) or originate from primary cortical cells (descending), *commissural* fibers arise from and terminate on association cells of the cerebral cortex. The major inter-hemispheric commissural connections are the corpus callosum, anterior commissure, and hippocampal commissure. (*Note:* The posterior commissure and habenular commissure

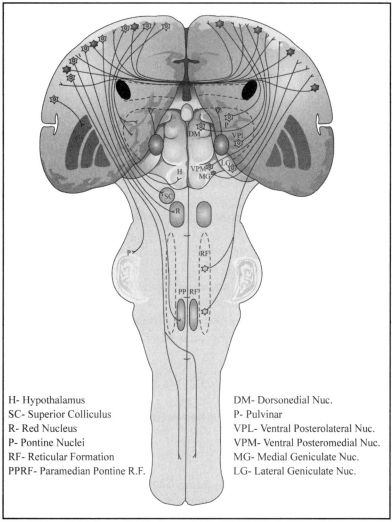

Figure 6-2: Schematic diagram of the organization of axons that form the subcortical white matter. Examples of ascending projections are illustrated on the right side of the diagram. Examples of descending projection bundles are illustrated on the left side of the diagram. An example of a commissural bundle is shown crossing between two hemispheres (Note: Association bundles are not illustrated in this figure.)

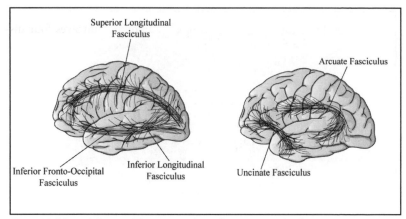

Figure 6-3: Schematic diagram of the major intra-hemispheric association bundles.

predominantly interconnect neural structures of the diencephalon and midbrain, and are thus technically not classified as inter-hemispheric commissural connections.)

13. Lesions involving the primary motor cortex affect motor performance. Lesions or disease processes involving primary sensory cortex typically affect perception of the modality in question. Lesions involving modality-specific association cortex typically affect the individual's ability to recognize the stimulus or the meaning of the stimulus, deficits referred to as *agnosia*. Lesions involving integrative association cortex are characterized by more complicated deficits of experience and behavior.

14. Lesions or disease processes involving axons of the subcortical white matter produce signs and symptoms that reflect how affected areas of the CNS function when disconnected from other parts. Some functions or behaviors are lost, while others are altered in specific ways.

LANGUAGE

Key Points

1. *Language* refers to a method of communication that employs symbols to represent objects and ideas. This method of communication requires mechanisms to both convey and receive symbolic information. These methods include primarily speaking and listening and writing and reading.

2. Speech and language are **not** synonymous terms. *Speaking* refers to the process of producing symbolic sounds and involves four distinct processes: respiration, phonation, resonation, and articulation. *Respiration* refers to the movement of air over the vocal folds, through the nasal and oropharynx, and out through the mouth and nose. *Phonation* refers to the process of creating compression and rarefaction waves as a result of air passing through the glottis. *Resonation* refers to the subtle "shaping" of the moving air as it passes through the oropharynx and nasopharynx (and associated air sinuses of the skull). *Articulation* refers to the final "shaping" of expelled air by muscles of the tongue, jaw, lips, teeth, and face. These processes are controlled by muscles innervated by lower motor neurons, which in turn are influenced by a variety of upper motor neuron-containing nuclei and cortical areas. Lesions involving any of these may result in disorders of speech, including dysphonia and dysarthria.

3. The two most commonly used language mechanisms are speaking/listening and writing/reading. The former uses symbols referred to as *phonemes*. The latter uses symbols know as *graphemes*.

4. Language function in humans is a cortical function involving predominantly the perisylvian cortices (cortical areas located both above and below the sylvian fissure) together with an important subcortical fiber pathway that interconnects these cortical areas. The cortical areas include the pars triangularis and pars opercularis of the inferior frontal gyrus (Broca's area), the angular and supramarginal gyri of the parietal lobe, and the posterior part of the superior temporal gyrus (Wernicke's area). The subcortical white fiber pathway that interconnects these two areas is referred to as the *arcuate fasciculus.*

5. Different aspects of language function appear to be distributed between the right and left hemispheres. Clinical experience has shown that lesions involving the perisylvian cortices and/or subcortical white on the left side typically result in impairment of propositional language function in approximately 95% of naturally right-handed individuals and 70% of left-handed persons. In contrast, perisylvian lesions on the right side commonly result in impairment of prosodic language function in 95% of naturally right-handed individuals and 70% of naturally left-handed persons. These data are frequently overgeneralized in statements such as, "The left hemisphere is dominant for language." A more correct statement would be, "The left hemisphere appears to play a dominant role in mediating the propositional components of language function, whereas the right hemisphere appears to be important in connection with prosodic elements of language function."

6. *Propositional language function* refers to the ability to produce and interpret words in the lexicon and to use the rules of grammar and syntax. Essentially, this is the ability to communicate effectively by talking and listening, and writing and reading. *Prosodic language function* refers to the ability to use rhythm, rate, volume, tempo, inflection, and pitch to influence meaning of language symbols and the ability to interpret specific meaning based on the speaker's use of rhythm, rate, volume, tempo, inflection, and pitch. Remember, information is conveyed not only by what is said (propositional communication) but also by how it is said (prosodic communication).

7. Normal language function requires the ability to both produce and correctly interpret graphemes and phonemes. With regard to language function using phonemes, lesions involving the perisylvian cortices on the side specialized for the propositional components of language function result in language abnormalities known collectively as *aphasia*. With regard to communication using graphemes, the corresponding deficits are referred to as *agraphia* (difficulty with writing, a production deficit) and *dyslexia* (difficulty with reading, an interpretation deficit).

8. Localized intrahemispheric lesions result in different types of language impairments. In the hemisphere specialized for propositional language, lesions involving the perisylvian cortices of the inferior frontal gyrus (Broca's area) result predominantly in deficits of language production. These patients are dysfluent and much effort is required to communicate. They may become frustrated or angry with their inability to communicate effectively. Lesions involving the inferior parietal and superior temporal perisylvian cortices (Wernicke's area) result predominantly in difficulties with language comprehension. These patients produce fluent speech that is frequently devoid of appropriate or contextual meaning. These patients have difficulty understanding what they hear or read. Both groups of patients have difficulty repeating simple, nonsensical phrases such as "No ifs, ands, or buts."

9. The perisylvian cortices receive arterial blood supply by way of branches of the middle cerebral artery. The superior branches perfuse the suprasylvian cortices including Broca's area, while the inferior branches perfuse in infrasylvian cortices including Wernicke's area.

10. *Aphasia* refers to an acquired disorder of language function.

11. The transcortical aphasias are fundamentally disconnection syndromes in which the perisylvian language areas are partially de-afferented. In transcortical motor aphasia, Broca's area is separated from the prefrontal cortices. In transcortical sensory aphasia, Wernicke's

area is separated from parietal, occipital, and posterior temporal cortices. The transcortical aphasias are distinguished from the fluent and dysfluent aphasias by the observation that repetition ability is relatively intact in the former conditions.

12. *Conduction aphasia* refers to an abnormality of language function characterized by difficulty repeating short strings of words in individuals in whom comprehension and fluency are comparatively intact. Conduction aphasia is most commonly observed in individuals with small, focal subcortical lesions that interrupt transmission in the arcuate fasciculus but spare Broca's and Wernicke's areas.

13. The clinical evaluation of language function typically includes an evaluation of fluency, comprehension, repetition, reading and writing, and word finding.

APRAXIA AND AGNOSIA

Key Points

1. The term *praxis* refers to the ability to plan and carry out motor behaviors. The neural apparatus required for this ability includes (from the "bottom up") an intact and functioning muscular system and peripheral nervous system, intact lower and upper motor neurons, normal cerebellum and basal nuclei function, and (important in the context of this topic) normally functioning cortical association cells that project to and influence cells of the primary motor, premotor, and supplementary motor areas of the cerebral cortex.

2. *Apraxia*, in the most general sense, refers to the inability to carry out motor behaviors on request that spontaneously can be performed adequately and with ease. Apraxia represents a disturbance in the formulation and/or execution of a motor plan in the absence of mental disease or disease involving the principal motor apparatus. Implied in this definition is that the motor systems (upper motor neurons, lower motor neurons, cerebellum, basal ganglia, and muscles) are intact. The apraxias, therefore, are disorders affecting cortical association cells that project to and influence cells in the primary motor, premotor, and supplementary areas of the brain. Apraxias are disorders of higher cortical function.

3. Apraxia can be observed in the upper limb, lower limb, trunk, and head (eyes, face, mouth, and tongue). However, apractic disorders are most easily identified and described in the upper limb mainly because of the extensive use of the upper limbs in activities of daily living.

4. Humans, unlike many animals, use a large variety of gestures and objects (tools) in everyday life. Gestures and movements used to convey meaning that do not use tools or objects, such as waving or shaking a fist, are referred to as *intransitive* movements. *Transitive* movements, in contrast, are movements that involve the use of an object or a tool, such as driving a nail with a hammer, drinking from a glass, eating with a fork, or opening a bottle with a bottle opener. Both types of movements require neural mechanisms for planning and execution in order to achieve the desired outcome.

5. Several types of apraxia have been described, the most common of which are ideational (conceptual) apraxia, ideomotor apraxia, dressing apraxia, and buccofacial apraxia. Because most activities of daily living involve objects, tools, or implements of some sort, apraxias are most commonly described in terms of transitive movements.

6. The term *ideational praxis* typically refers to the general understanding of what tools are for, how they work, and how to select the right tool for an intended task. Ideational praxis involves the ability to decide, based on available information, which tool might be required for a particular purpose. It involves the ability to select a substitute tool for a job in the event that a better tool is unavailable.

7. Ideational apraxia is characterized by the inability to select a tool or object needed for a particular task. Given a task such as screwing a screw into a board, the individual may either pick an inappropriate tool such as a file or may pick no tool at all and attempt to twist the screw with his or her fingers or pound it with his or her hand. Ideational apraxia is seen in association with lesions involving the superior parietal lobule on the left side, affecting cortical cells that project axons to the motor cortices of the frontal lobe by way of the superior longitudinal fasciculus. Ideational apraxia is not uncommon in patients with Alzheimer's disease.

8. The term *ideomotor praxis* refers to the ability to properly use the correct or best tool for a particular task. It reflects a correct understanding about what tools are used for and the basic principles underlying their operation and use.

9. Ideomotor apraxia is characterized by the inability to properly complete a task using a tool after having successfully selected the appropriate tool. Individuals with ideomotor apraxia understand the requirements of the tool-requiring task but are unable to perform the task. It is as if they have forgotten how to use a fork, a hammer, or a toothbrush for their intended purposes. On clinical examination, such patients may be unable to perform simple, multiple-step tasks.

For example, the individual will fail upon request to fold a piece of paper twice, place it in an envelope, and then place the envelope on the floor. In terms of intransitive movements, individuals with ideomotor apraxia will not be able to demonstrate upon request how to "wave goodbye" or give the "thumbs up sign." Interestingly, neither transitive nor intransitive tasks can be performed in a pantomime fashion, suggesting that even though the individual can see the task performed, they are nonetheless unable to organize motor commands needed to carry out the movement(s). Ideomotor apraxia is seen in association with lesions involving the parieto-occipital area of the left side, affecting cells that project axons to the motor cortices by way of the superior longitudinal fasciculus. In patients with ideomotor apraxia, intransitive movements tend to be less affected than transitive movements.

10. *Dressing praxis* refers to the ability to properly clothe oneself. It involves an understanding of the structure of various garments, how they are manipulated to cover the body, and how a variety of movements involving multiple body parts (limbs) are sequenced in order to properly don the particular piece of apparel (shirt, pants, socks, shoes). Dressing apraxia is characterized by difficulty or the inability to dress properly and is seen in association with lesions involving the parietal lobe on the right side.

11. *Buccofacial praxis* refers to the ability to perform movements using the muscles innervated by the cranial nerves (extraocular muscles, muscles of mastication and facial expression, pharynx, and tongue). While many of these movements are automatic, others such as puckering the lips, sticking out the tongue, sucking on a straw, and swallowing can be performed upon request and therefore can be affected by lesions involving certain regions of the cerebral cortex. Buccofacial apraxia is characterized by the impaired ability to properly perform the above-mentioned actions, either upon request or in pantomime. Buccofacial apraxia is most commonly seen in association with lesions involving the inferior frontal gyrus and insula on the left side. These areas are the origin of projections to the rather large "face" area of the precentral gyrus (primary motor cortex).

12. The term *gnosis* refers to the ability to recognize based on perceived characteristics. Gnosis is further classified according to the sensory modality involved. Thus we can refer to visual gnosis, tactile gnosis, auditory gnosis, olfactory gnosis, and gustatory gnosis.

13. *Agnosia* refers to the inability to recognize a perceived stimulus. Agnosia implies that the stimulus is perceived, that it is experienced, but that it is not recognized as what it is. As a result, the object cannot

be named based on that particular modality, but can be identified and named using another modality. Agnosia implies that the functions of the structures involved in stimulus transduction, transmission, and perception are intact, but that areas of the cerebral cortex required for interpretation are either damaged or disconnected from the primary cortical areas. While the ability to interpret any of the sensory modalities can become impaired, most agnosias in humans involve the visual system.

14. *Visual agnosia* refers to a failure to recognize objects based on their visual characteristics, with preserved recognition using another sensory modality in the absence of impaired primary visual perception. Two types of visual agnosia are commonly described: apperceptive agnosia and associative agnosia.

15. *Apperceptive agnosia* is characterized by an inability to assemble visualized stimuli (typically edges, contours, colors) into a coherent mental representation of an object. (For example, shown a picture of a pair of spectacles, the subject may say that he sees a bicycle.) If the same object is viewed from two different perspectives, it will be experienced as two different objects. Individuals with apperceptive agnosia are unable to draw familiar objects or match different pictures of the same object. Apperceptive agnosia is seen in individuals with bilateral lesions involving the occipital lobes.

16. *Associative agnosia* is characterized as an inability to recognize and name objects based on their visual features. However, unlike apperceptive agnosia, individuals with associative agnosia are able to draw objects presented to them and are able to match similar objects. The deficit here is an inability to recognize and name the object based on visual cues. Associative agnosia is seen in individuals with lesions involving the parieto-occipital area on the left side.

17. *Prosopagnosia* is a specific form of agnosia characterized by an inability to recognize individuals by their face. Individuals with prosopagnosia, while unable to identify persons by face, are typically able to identify them by their voice, touch, and even by their gait pattern from a distance. Prosopagnosia is seen in individuals with lesions involving the parieto-occipital areas on the right side.

18. Clinical evidence suggests that recognition may not be based on only experiential data, but also have emotional components. For example, visual stimuli may elicit simple perceptual recognition as well as evoke strong emotional responses. These two effects may reflect transmission from the visual association cortices on the right side to two separate structures in the right temporal lobe. Simple recognition

based on memory may involve projections from the visual association cortices to the hippocampus via the *ventral pathway* of the inferior longitudinal fasciculus, while the emotional component of visual recognition may be mediated via projections to the amygdaloid complex by way of the *dorsal pathway* of the inferior longitudinal fasciculus. These two components of visual recognition may be dissociated in patients with small, focal lesions affecting only one of the two above-mentioned pathways.

CONSCIOUSNESS

Key Points

1. *Consciousness* refers to the ability of an individual to experience and respond to a variety of endogenous and exogenous stimuli. This ability is thought to be a function of particular groups of neurons in the brainstem and forebrain as suggested by the clinical observation that disease or injury involving these parts of the CNS is frequently associated with specific forms of altered consciousness.

2. An individual's state of consciousness at any point in time is subject to change. Changes occur in neurologically intact individuals, such as when an individual shifts from the waking state to the sleeping state. Changes in consciousness from the waking state to the sleep state are the result of normal physiological processes. Alterations in consciousness can also be the result of pathological processes, as exemplified by abnormal states such as lethargy, obtundation, stupor, and coma.

3. From an evaluative point of view, consciousness is thought to consist of two components: arousal (level of consciousness) and awareness (content of consciousness). *Arousal* refers to a primitive set of automatic reflex responses involving a phylogenetically old, diffusely distributed network of nuclei and pathways located in the diencephalon and brainstem reticular formation. Collectively, these nuclei and pathways comprise what is commonly referred to as the *ascending reticular activating system* (ARAS). *Awareness* refers to the integration of multiple sensory experiences that result in a meaningful and authentic understanding of the environment and the self. The anatomical substrate of awareness is the cerebral cortex.

4. Pathological alterations in arousal are suggestive of brainstem dysfunction. Decreased states of arousal are commonly marked by abnormalities of brainstem and spinal-mediated reflex functions. Common causes of decreased arousal include direct trauma to the

brainstem, vascular events (usually hemorrhage) in the brainstem, and brainstem compression/displacement, frequently associated with rapid increases in intracranial pressure.

5. Disease-related alterations in awareness are frequently marked by changes in mental status, particularly delirium, confusion, and abnormalities in cognitive function. Altered states of awareness are commonly associated with toxic and metabolic insults to the brain. Delirium, in particular, is not uncommon in hospitalized individuals and the elderly.

6. Consciousness can be evaluated in several different ways. Perhaps the most commonly used assessment tool is the Glasgow Coma Scale (GCS). The evaluation includes quantitative measures of eye opening, best motor response to verbal or tactile stimuli, and best verbal response to auditory stimuli. Scores range from 3 (unconscious) to 15 (conscious). Other, more detailed examination techniques may be used to evaluate specific aspects of either level of consciousness or content of consciousness.

LIMBIC SYSTEM

Key Points

1. The *limbic system* in humans is a functional system concerned primarily with how individuals feel and how they act and behave in connection with those feelings. The system plays a role in adaptive behavior and behavior aimed at achieving personal wants and needs.

2. The two central anatomical structures of the limbic system are the amygdaloid nucleus and the hippocampal formation. The *amygdaloid nucleus* is involved in determining and shaping specific reactions (autonomic, somatic motor, and endocrine) and overall behavior in response to stimuli, thoughts, events, and experiences that are personally and emotionally significant. The *hippocampal formation* is involved in processes associated with learning and remembering.

3. The amygdaloid nucleus (amygdala) is located in the anterior part of the temporal lobe. It is reciprocally interconnected with nuclei of the brainstem, thalamus, and hypothalamus and with widespread areas of the cerebral cortex. Most of the input to the amygdala originates in the cerebral cortex including the olfactory bulb. Projections from the amygdala are directed largely to the hypothalamus for regulation of autonomic and endocrine effects and to the cerebral cortex through the thalamus for regulation of somatic motor behaviors. The behaviors

affected are sometimes described as *drive-related* and *emotion-related*. Drive-related behaviors are aimed at attaining goals related to individual wants (I want this), while emotion-related behaviors are aimed at attaining goals related to perceived threats (survival behaviors) and individual needs (I need this). Stimulation of the amygdala in humans is associated with feelings of fear, confusion, disturbances of awareness, and amnesia for events occurring during stimulation. Lesions involving the amygdala in humans have been reported to result in a reduction in aggressive and assaultive behavior.

4. The hippocampal formation is a phylogenetically old cortical structure that is involved in the conversion of experiences, perceptions, and thoughts into memories. The ability to form retrievable memories provides for limited thinking and behavioral choice in adapting to a changing environment. Access to memories regarding past experiences (or more likely, the consequences of exposure to a stimulus, situation, or occurrence in the past), permits the individual to possibly change (eliminate, modify, or enhance) a particular behavioral response or reaction when that stimulus or situation is encountered again. When the reaction or response to an encounter with a previously experienced stimulus or situation is different from the initial reaction or response, learning is said to have occurred.

5. The hippocampal formation consists of the dentate gyrus, hippocampus, and subiculum (Figure 6-4). Synaptic input to the hippocampal formation is derived largely from the entorhinal cortex of the medial and ventral temporal lobe. The output of the hippocampal formation is by way of the fornix, which terminates largely in the septal area (nuclei), hypothalamus (mammillary nucleus), and thalamus (anterior and dorsal medial nuclei).

6. Among the important connections within the limbic system is the Papez circuit. The Papez circuit is a loop pathway involving the hippocampal formation, mamillary nucleus, anterior nucleus of the thalamus, and the cingulate gyrus.

7. Certain cells in the hippocampal formation, specifically cells in the CA1 region of the hippocampus (Sommer's sector), are unusually sensitive to hypoxia, such as might occur in patients who suffer cardiac arrest. Memory deficits sometimes seen in patients who survive cardiac arrest are thought to be related to hypoxia-induced cell damage to cells in Sommer's sector.

8. Some cells in the hippocampal formation bear a class of glutamate receptors known as *NMDA receptors*. These receptors have been shown to be involved in the process of *long-term potentiation* (LTP), a process functionally associated with memory formation.

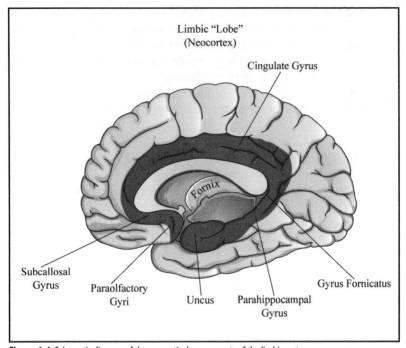

Figure 6-4: Schematic diagram of the neocortical components of the limbic system.

9. Several different classification systems have been developed to describe and help understand the processes and neural mechanisms involved in learning and remembering. One such scheme divides the processes of learning and remembering into three component processes. *Acquisition* refers to the process of entering information into consciousness. *Consolidation* refers to the process of creating and storing memories of the experience. *Retrieval* refers to the process of calling back into consciousness some features or aspects about the information previously learned. Each of these processes is associated with specific neuronal processes and system activity, with some being better understood than others.

10. For clinical purposes, learning and remembering are frequently divided into three components, each of which can be assessed and evaluated on clinical examination. *Immediate recall*, sometimes referred to as working memory, refers to the ability to recall or maintain awareness of information encountered several seconds earlier,

typically without an intervening distraction. The major requirements for immediate recall are the conscious state and the neurological ability to attend (attention) to the information to be remembered. *Short-term memory*, sometimes referred to as recent memory, refers to the ability to retrieve and recall information encountered (learned) minutes to hours earlier, typically with an intervening distraction such as shifting attention to other, generally unrelated types of information. The major requirements for short-term memory formation are neuronal protein synthesis and neuronal activation in new patterns as a result of the information or experience. NMDA receptor bearing cells in the hippocampal formation and LTP are implicated in the process of short-term memory formation. *Long-term memory* refers to the ability to retrieve and recall information encountered (learned) months to years previously. The major requirement for long-term memory formation is synaptic reorganization in the cerebral cortex resulting from neuronal activity associated with the learning process. On a neuronal level, learning-induced changes in the synaptic profile of a cell mean that the cell will, as a result of these changes, receive different synaptic input from its afferent sources and respond differently to those inputs.

11. Memory is alternatively classified as procedural or declarative. *Procedural memory* (implicit memory) refers to the ability to remember how to perform certain actions or activities learned in the past, such as riding a bicycle. It may also refer to the ability to remember how to perform certain mental activities, such as how to use information and strategies to create or solve problems. *Declarative memory* (explicit memory) refers to the ability to remember facts, faces, names, events, and similar types of information. Declarative memory is sometimes divided into *episodic* and *semantic* categories, with episodic memory referring to information remembered in relation to a particular situation or context, such as the names of the US presidents, and semantic memory referring to verbal and pictorial information remembered, even though we no longer remember where or how we learned it.

12. Memories previously formed that cannot be retrieved at will are not necessarily lost (forgotten). They may rather be rendered inaccessible by some mechanism (ie, distraction) but can be retrieved by certain commonly used methods (ie, cuing, organizing). The ability to bring into consciousness (remember) experiences from the past indicates that learning occurred when the past experience was part of the present.

13. An individual's identity is molded and shaped on a continual basis by the ability to learn and remember events, people, and experiences from the past.

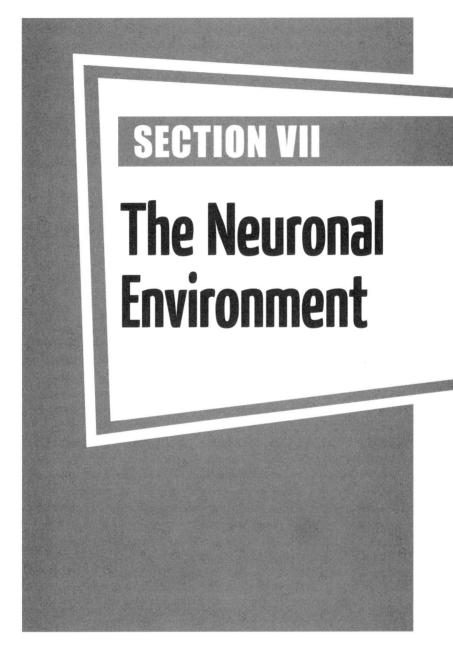

SECTION VII

The Neuronal Environment

Nolan M.
Cram Session in Functional Neuroanatomy:
A Handbook for Students & Clinicians (pp. 189-212)
© 2012 SLACK Incorporated

MENINGES AND DURAL VENOUS SINUSES

Key Points

1. The central nervous system (CNS) (brain and spinal cord) is enclosed within three layers of connective tissue referred to as the *meninges*. The cranial meninges line the inside of the cranial vault and compartmentalize the intracranial space. The spinal meninges surround the spinal cord and help to secure the spinal cord within the vertebral canal.

2. The outermost layer of the meninges is the *dura mater*. Because of its relative thickness, it is sometimes referred to as the *pachymeninx*. This layer, formed by fibroblasts and collagen fibers, derives its blood supply from meningeal arteries, where it surrounds the brain within the cranial cavity, and from segmental spinal arteries, where it surrounds the spinal cord within the vertebral canal.

3. Within the cranium, the dura mater consists of two layers: an endosteal (periosteal) layer and meningeal (falx) layer (Figure 7-1). The *endosteal* layer, the more superficial of the two dural layers, lines the cranial cavity and is firmly attached to the innermost layer of the skull. It is particularly adherent in the region of the suture lines. The *meningeal* (falx) layer, the deeper of the two layers, separates the cranial cavity into smaller compartments and supports the posterior regions of the cerebral hemispheres. Where the meningeal layer separates from the endosteal layer, distinct anatomical structures are formed known as the *falx cerebri, falx cerebelli, tentorium cerebelli,* and *diaphragma sellae*. These dural structures compartmentalize the cranial cavity and mark the location of certain dural venous sinuses. The tentorium cerebelli divides the cranial cavity into two separate regions, the *supratentorial* compartment located above the tentorium cerebelli, which contains the cerebral hemispheres and thalamus, and the *infratentorial* compartment located below the tentorium in which is found the brainstem and cerebellum. The cranial dura does not extend into any of the fissures or sulci of the brain. The intracranial dura mater receives sensory innervation by way of branches of the trigeminal nerve.

4. In regions where the endosteal and meningeal layers separate, valveless endothelial-lined channels are formed known as *dural venous sinuses*. The dural venous sinuses receive unoxygenated blood from veins draining the cerebrum, cerebellum, and brainstem. Blood flows through the dural venous sinuses to drain from the cranial cavity into

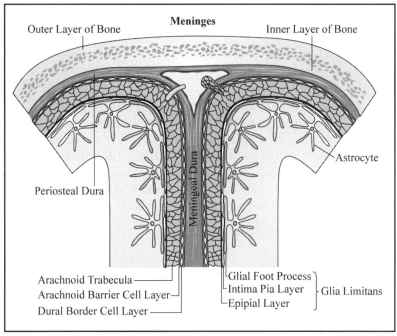

Figure 7-1: Schematic diagram of the organization of the intracranial meninges.

the internal jugular veins. Because of their location in the margins of the dura mater, dural venous sinuses are essentially incompressible and will remain patent in the presence of increased *intracranial pressure* (ICP).

5. Histologically, two distinct, clinically important regions of the dural layer are recognized. The more superficial region of both the endosteal and meningeal layers is formed by fibroblasts and collagen fibers. The collagen fibers provide structural stability to these layers of the dura mater. The deeper region, known as the *dural border cell layer,* is formed by fibroblasts but lacks the collagen fibers found in the more superficial layer. As a result, intercellular junctions in this layer are less strong and the cells (fibroblasts) are more easily separated by mechanical and other forces that may be produced by disease or injury.

6. Within the vertebral canal, the dura mater is separated from the spinal cord by a space (epidural space) that contains fat and an epidural plexus of veins. It is composed of layers of fibroblasts and collagen

fibers. The dura mater exists as a tubular structure that extends from the level of the foramen magnum to the S2 vertebral segment, where it tapers into a single strand called the *coccygeal ligament* (sometimes known as the *filum terminale externum*) and extends caudally to attach to the coccyx.

7. The intermediate layer of the meninges, the *arachnoid mater*, is also composed of fibroblasts and collagen fibers. Although the overall layer is much thinner than the dura, the cells of this layer are joined by tight junctions, resulting in the formation of a watertight membrane surrounding the brain and spinal cord. The intracranial arachnoid membrane is tightly adherent to the overlying dura mater and like the dura, does not extend into the cerebral fissures or sulci. The arachnoid membrane is attached to the more deeply located pia mater by way of thread-like structures known as *arachnoid trabeculae*. The space formed between the arachnoid above and the pia mater below is referred to as the *subarachnoid space*. The subarachnoid space contains cerebrospinal fluid together with a network of extracerebral arteries and veins. At certain locations, the subarachnoid space is relatively large. These enlarged regions are known as *cisterns*.

8. The arachnoid layer within the vertebral canal lies closely opposed to the deep surface of the spinal dura and like the dura, exists as a tubular structure that extends caudally from the level of the foramen magnum to the S2 vertebral segment. There it tapers into a single strand that becomes incorporated into the coccygeal ligament. The subarachnoid space located between the caudal tip of the spinal cord (*conus medullaris*) located approximately at the level of the L1-L2 intervertebral disc and the S2 vertebra level is commonly referred to as the *lumbar cistern*.

9. Arachnoid granulations are specialized structures found in close proximity to dural venous sinuses and near dorsal root ganglia. These structures function as one-way valves that permit *cerebrospinal fluid* (CSF) to pass from the subarachnoid space into the dural venous sinuses or into the small veins near dorsal root ganglia.

10. The pia mater consists of two embryologically and histologically distinct layers: the *epipial layer* (a more superficial, mesodermal-derived layer composed of fibroblasts and collagen fibers), and the *intima pial layer* (a deeper, ectodermal-derived layer composed of reticular and elastic fibers). In the spinal canal, the epipial layer gives rise to structures referred to as *denticulate ligaments* that extend laterally to attach to the dural layer. These structures help to anchor the spinal cord within the meningeal envelope. In the region of the anterior median fissure, the spinal pia mater is thickened to form the *linea*

splendens, a connective tissue structure along which passes penetrating branches of the anterior spinal artery. The term *leptomeninges* refers to the combined arachnoid mater and pia mater, specifically the arachnoid and epipial layer of pia mater.

11. The intima pia lies superficial to and in direct contact with cytoplasmic extensions (foot processes) of glial cells (astrocytes) throughout the CNS. This barrier is referred to as the *glia-limitans.* The cells forming the glia-limitans are not joined by tight junctions, thus the glia-limitans is not a watertight barrier.

12. A fluid-filled space exists between the arachnoid mater and pia mater known as the *subarachnoid space.* This space, surrounding both the brain and spinal cord, contains CSF. Comparatively large regions of subarachnoid space are referred to as *cisterns.* Most of the CSF in the cranial cavity is located in these subarachnoid cisterns. Most of the CSF in the vertebral canal is located in the lumbar cistern, the location from which CSF can be sampled by means of lumbar puncture.

13. In addition to CSF, the intracranial subarachnoid space contains an extensive plexus of arteries and arterioles, the so-called *meningeal anastomosis* or *meningeal plexus.* These vessels form a superficial network of vessels that give rise to the smaller, penetrating vessels of the brain.

14. Injury to blood vessels in relation to the meninges can occur from a variety of causes. Collections of extravasated blood (hematoma) are frequently described using terms indicating their location with respect to the meninges. Thus, intracranial, extracerebral hematomas are said to be *epidural, subdural,* or *subarachnoid* in location. Each type of hematoma can be characterized by features as its etiologic mechanism, natural course, and clinical outcome. Epidural hemorrhage is seen most frequently in young adult populations and is commonly associated with rather severe head trauma that results in damage to one of the meningeal arteries—most frequently, the middle meningeal artery in the region of the pterion. Blood passes out of the injured vessel under arterial pressure and accumulates by dissection within the superficial layers of the dura. Subdural hemorrhage is most frequently seen in elderly individuals and is commonly associated with relatively mild head trauma that results in damage by stretching of the delicate bridging veins as they course from the surface of the brain to the dural venous sinuses. Blood passes out of the injured vessel under venous pressure and accumulates by dissecting within the dural border cell layer, immediately superficial to the arachnoid membrane. Subarachnoid hemorrhage is seen in both the adult and elderly populations and is associated with bleeding from aneurysms

and *arteriovenous malformations* (AVM) involving vessels lying in the subarachnoid space surrounding the brain.

ARTERIAL BLOOD SUPPLY

Key Points

1. The brain receives approximately 15% to 20% of resting cardiac output, amounting to approximately 750 to 800 milliliters of blood per minute. This volume of blood is required to deliver sufficient quantities of glucose and oxygen to satisfy the comparatively high metabolic demands of the brain.

2. Arterial blood is delivered to the brain chiefly by way of the internal carotid artery and its branches (anterior circulation) and the vertebral and basilar arteries and their branches (posterior circulation). In the hemodynamically symmetrical individual, approximately 70±10% of the total blood flow to the brain (approximately 525 mL/min) is delivered by way of the anterior circulation, with 30±10% (225 mL/min) being delivered by way of the posterior circulation. The two circulatory systems are connected at the base of the brain by way of the posterior communicating artery.

3. The *internal carotid artery* (ICA) arises at approximately the C4 vertebral level as one of two terminal branches of the common carotid artery. The ICA ascends in the neck within the carotid sheath, passes through the base of the skull and the cavernous sinus to enter the middle cranial fossa, where it terminates immediately lateral to the optic chiasm by bifurcating to form the *middle cerebral artery* (MCA) and the *anterior cerebral artery* (ACA). The ICA is divided into seven parts or segments: *cervical* (C1), *petrous* (C2), *lacerum* (C3), *cavernous* (C4), *clinoid* (C5), *ophthalmic* (C6), and *communicating* (C7).

4. The ICAs and their branches (anterior circulation) perfuse brain structures of the supratentorial compartment, including the frontal and parietal lobes and underlying gray and white matter, the lateral surface of the occipital lobe, the superior part of the temporal lobe, the anterior regions of the basal nuclei, and the anterior regions of the internal capsule. The major intracranial branches of the internal carotid artery, in addition to its two terminal branches (MCA and ACA), are the ophthalmic artery, the posterior communicating artery, and the anterior choroidal artery.

5. The *ophthalmic artery* arises from the ophthalmic segment of the ICA and passes anteriorly through the optic canal together with

the optic nerve. The ophthalmic artery supplies the eye, optic nerve, extraocular muscles, and related intraorbital structures. Branches of the ophthalmic artery form important anastomotic connections within the orbit with branches of the external carotid artery.

6. The *posterior communicating artery* (PComA) arises slightly distal to the ophthalmic artery and lies superior to the cavernous sinus. This artery interconnects the ICA with the *posterior cerebral artery* (PCA) and forms an important anastomotic connection between the anterior circulation and the posterior circulation. (*Note*: In the fetus, the developing occipital lobe is perfused by the PCA supplied by the ICA by way of the PComA. In the adult, this area of the brain is perfused primarily by way of the PCA supplied by the basilar artery.)

7. The *anterior choroidal artery* (AChA) arises slightly distal to the PComA and courses in a posteromedial direction lying at first medial to the ICA, then along the inferior surface of the optic tract. The artery passes through the choroidal fissure to supply the choroid plexus of the lateral ventricle. In addition to perfusing the choroid plexus, the AChA supplies the optic tract and lateral geniculate body, hippocampus including the uncus, globus pallidus, and the posterior part of the posterior limb of the internal capsule.

8. The two terminal branches of the ICA are the MCA and the ACA. In the hemodynamically symmetrical individual, approximately 80±10% of the blood delivered to the bifurcation passes into the MCA, with the remaining 20±10% passing into the ACA.

9. The MCA, the larger of the two terminal branches, arises as a single branch lateral to the optic chiasm and courses laterally toward the insula. The MCA is commonly divided into four segments: *sphenoidal* (M1), *insular* (M2), *opercular* (M3), and *cortical* (M4).

10. The M1 segment arises at the bifurcation of the ICA and courses laterally through the sphenoidal cistern toward the insular cortex. It frequently divides into two branches, a superior trunk and inferior trunk, before reaching the insula. The M1 segment gives rise to several penetrating branches (lenticulostriate arteries) that pass superiorly through the anterior perforated space to supply the anterior part of the corpus striatum and internal capsule.

11. The M2 segment lies on the lateral surface of and supplies the insular cortex and underlying white matter.

12. The M3 segment lies on the deep surface of the frontal and parietal opercula above and temporal opercula below, extending from the circular sulcus to the lateral fissure. Branches of this segment supply the medial cortical surfaces of the operculum and underlying white matter.

13. The M4 segment consists of as many as 12 branches located largely in the subarachnoid space on the lateral surface of the cerebral hemisphere. These branches give rise to penetrating arteries that supply the cortical surface together with the superficial parts of the underlying subcortical white matter. These vessels establish important anastomotic connections with cortical branches of the ACA and PCA, forming *watershed zones.*

14. The ACA is the smaller of the two terminal branches of the ICA. The artery passes anteromedially toward the interhemispheric fissure, passing above the optic nerve. The artery then courses anteriorly, beneath the rostrum of the corpus callosum, superiorly in front of the genu, and posteriorly on the superior surface of the corpus callosum, extending toward the splenium. The ACA ends as a small branch in the choroid plexus in the roof of the third ventricle. The ACA is divided into five segments: *precommunicating* (A1), *infracallosal* (A2), *precallosal* (A3), *supracallosal* (A4), and *postcallosal* (A5). Frequently, the A2-A5 segments are collectively referred to as the *pericallosal artery.* The two ACAs are interconnected immediately in front of the lamina terminalis by a small artery called the *anterior communicating artery* (AComA). The ACA gives rise to penetrating branches that supply deep structure in the anterior part of the brain, including the anterior part of the corpus striatum, anterior limb of the internal capsule, columns of the fornix, septal nuclei, anterior commissure, and corpus callosum, and to cortical braches that supply the orbital cortex and medial surface of the frontal and parietal lobes, including the cingulate gyrus.

15. The posterior circulation consists of the vertebral and basilar arteries and their branches. These vessels supply structures located in the infratentorial compartment of the cranial vault, including the brainstem and cerebellum as well as structures located in the supratentorial compartment, including gyri on the medial surface of the occipital and temporal lobes and the posterior regions of the thalamus and internal capsule. The major branches of the vertebrobasilar vessels are the *anterior* and *posterior spinal arteries,* the *posterior inferior cerebellar artery,* the *anterior inferior cerebellar artery,* the *paramedian* and *short circumferential branches of the basilar artery,* the *labyrinthine artery,* and the *superior cerebellar artery.* The basilar artery terminates near the ponto-mesencephalic junction by bifurcating to form the posterior cerebral arteries.

16. The vertebral artery (VA) extends from the subclavian artery to the level of the pontomedullary junction of the brainstem. The artery is divided into extradural and intradural segments, each of which

is further divided into smaller segments. The extradural part of the VA extends from the origin from the subclavian artery to essentially where it enters the infratentorial compartment through the foramen magnum. The intradural part extends from the level of the foramen magnum to the pontomesenephalic junction where the vessel bifurcates forming its terminal branches. The extradural segment is further divided into three smaller segments: *prevertebral* (V1), *cervical* (V2), and *atlantic* (V3). The intradural segment (V4) is divided into two segments: *lateral medullary* and *anterior medullary*.

17. The *anterior spinal arteries* (ASAs) commonly arise from the intradural segment of the vertebral artery. These vessels course inferiorly along the ventrolateral surface of the medulla oblongata to fuse in the midline above the pyramidal decussation. Caudal to the point of fusion, the now unpaired, single anterior spinal artery lies in the ventromedian fissure and gives rise to penetrating branches that supply the medullary pyramids, medial lemniscus, and hypoglossal nuclei. The anterior spinal artery continues caudally throughout the length of the spinal cord, receiving branches the spinal vasocorona. The *posterior spinal arteries* (PSA) may arise from either the atlantic (V3) segment of the extradural part of the VA or the *posterior inferior cerebellar artery* (PICA). The arteries lie on the dorsolateral surface of the spinal cord near the emerging dorsal rootlets and supply the dorsal funiculus, dorsal horn, and dorsolateral part of the lateral funiculus.

18. The *posterior inferior cerebellar artery* (PICA) commonly arises from the intradural segment of the vertebral artery. The vessel takes a tortuous course, passing along the lateral surface of the medulla oblongata to reach the cerebellum, where its branches supply the posterior inferior parts of the cerebellum. Importantly, penetrating branches of the PICA supply structures located in the lateral part of the rostral half of the medulla oblongata, including the spinal lemniscus, spinal nucleus and tract of the trigeminal nerve, inferior cerebellar peduncle, and descending reticulospinal tracts terminating in the intermediolateral nucleus of the spinal cord.

19. The *anterior inferior cerebellar artery* (AICA) most commonly arises from the caudal part of the basilar artery. The AICA courses laterally toward the cerebellopontine angle, passing in close relationship to the facial and vestibulocochlear nerves. The artery continues onto the surface of the cerebellum, terminating in branches that ramify on the flocculus and the petrosal surface. Along its course, it gives rise to penetrating branches that supply structures in the lateral region of the caudal part of the pons, as well as the facial and vestibulocochlear nerves and the choroid plexus of the fourth ventricle.

20. The paramedian and short circumferential branches of the basilar artery penetrate the pons from its ventral surface to supply the pontine nuclei, longitudinal pontine fibers, abducens nucleus, and other nuclei and long ascending and descending pathways located in the pontine tegmentum.

21. The *superior cerebellar artery* (SCA) arises from the rostral part of the basilar artery immediately below its terminal bifurcation. The artery courses laterally around the brainstem at the pontomesencephalic junction to reach the cerebellomesencephalic fissure, where it divides into several cortical branches that ramify on the superior (tentorial) surface of the cerebellum. Perforating branches supply structures of the rostral part of the midbrain and cerebellum, including the superior cerebellar peduncle and the deep cerebellar nuclei.

22. The *posterior cerebral artery* (PCA) arises from the bifurcation of the basilar artery in the anterior midline at the level of the pontomesencephalic junction. The artery courses laterally around the midbrain in the crural and ambient cisterns and passes upward through the tentorial incisura to terminate in branches that lie on the medial surface of the occipital lobe and medial part of the inferior surface of the temporal lobe. Branches of the PCA supply regions of the midbrain, posterior part of the thalamus, hypothalamus, and choroid plexus of the third ventricle as well as cortical areas of the occipital and temporal lobes. The PCA is divided into four segments: precommunicating (P1), lateral cisternal (P2), quadrigeminal (P3), and cortical (P4).

23. The anterior and posterior circulations are interconnected by way of the posterior communicating artery, an anastomotic connection that becomes functionally important in individuals who develop certain types of occlusive cerebrovascular disease. The posterior communicating arteries, together with branches of the anterior and posterior cerebral arteries, form an important anastomotic network in the region of the hypothalamus known as the *circle of Willis*. Autopsy and imaging studies reveal that the circle of Willis is symmetrical (ie, it looks like illustrations in textbooks and atlases) in approximately 30% to 40% of individuals. Asymmetry or even the congenital absence of a part of the circle of Willis is thus not uncommon and does not, in and of itself, result in the development of neurologic signs or symptoms.

24. The circle of Willis is a ring-like or diamond-shaped anastomotic network of vessels occupying the basal cistern located at the base of the brain, below the hypothalamus. The circle of Willis is formed by the AComA and the A1 segments of the ACAs anteriorly and the two PComAs and the two P1 segments of the PCAs posteriorly. The ring-like structure is completed on each side by the choroidal segment of

the ICA. The functional significance of the circle of Willis lies in the fact that, in the extreme, should three or fewer of the four vessels that deliver blood to the brain become occluded, blood delivered by the remaining vessel could be delivered to all branches of the occluded vessel distal to the occlusion. However, in a more practical sense, vascular disease processes and various anatomical variations involving different parts of the circle of Willis, several of which will be summarized below, frequently limit the effectiveness of the anastomotic channels in preventing hypoperfusion-related neuronal injury.

25. Most anatomical diagrams depict the circle of Willis as symmetrical bilaterally. However, in reality, the circle is asymmetric in as many as 80% of the individuals or specimens studied. Anatomical variations include components that are absent, small in size (*hypoplastic*), or in some cases duplicate or multiple. Individual components of the circle of Willis may be patent or not patent (*atretic*). The normal response to any of these variations includes a compensatory increase in the size of the other components of the circle, further contributing to the observed asymmetry. So, although anatomical asymmetry is the rule rather than the exception, compensatory mechanisms, both anatomical and physiological, operate to prevent or at least reduce the likelihood of the individual experiencing signs and symptoms secondary to brain hypoperfusion.

26. Three functionally important anastomotic networks exist to help assure adequate blood delivery to the brain when flow is reduced or obstructed in one or more of the four major vessels that supply the brain. These are 1) the anastomotic connection between the internal carotid and vertebrobasilar vessels by way of the posterior communicating arteries, 2) connections between the internal carotid and external carotid vessels by way of the ophthalmic artery as well as several other vessels of lesser prominence, and 3) anastomotic connections between branches of the cerebral arteries in the intracranial subarachnoid space on the surface of the brain, the so called *meningeal anastomosis* or *plexuses*. In disease conditions in which a particular vessel or vessels become occluded, anastomotic networks allow blood to be delivered from areas with adequate and intact flow to areas with reduced blood flow. Remember, hemodynamically, blood will always flow down a pressure gradient.

27. Two morphologically distinct types of capillaries are found in the brain. In certain areas, collectively known as the *circumventricular organs*, the capillaries are characterized by fenestrae. The capillary beds in these regions of the brain permit the free movement by diffusion of ions and a variety of macromolecules down their concentration

gradients, both into and out of the vascular lumen. Nerve cells that comprise the circumventricular organs are thus affected by, and can respond to, alterations in the composition and concentration of substances in the blood. Likewise, substances synthesized and released by these cells can easily enter the bloodstream at these sites.

28. The majority of the capillaries in the CNS are lined by endothelial cells that are joined by tight junctions, membrane structures that effectively prevent the intercellular movement of substances between the vascular and extracellular compartments of the brain. Thus, in most regions of the brain, most substances must pass through the capillary endothelial cells, passing through both luminal and abluminal cell membranes as well as the endothelial cell cytoplasm, in order to reach nerve cells and glial cells. Some substances move across the endothelial cell membranes by diffusion, while others depend on energy-requiring pump mechanisms and carrier-mediated transport systems. Most substances, particularly large molecular weight substances, are unable to enter the brain by way of the vascular system. This barrier system, which consists of both structural (endothelial tight junctions) and physiological (diffusional and energy requiring transport systems) components, is referred to as the *blood-brain barrier* (BBB).

REGULATION OF CEREBRAL BLOOD FLOW

Key Points

1. The brain receives a disproportionately large blood supply for its size, amounting to approximately 20% of resting cardiac output. *Cerebral blood flow* (CBF) in the resting state is approximately 750 ml/min. This volume of blood is necessary to deliver sufficient oxygen and glucose to meet the high energy demands of the brain. In the resting state, the brain requires approximately 50 ml of oxygen to metabolize approximately 75 mg of glucose per minute.

2. Blood is delivered to the brain by way of the internal carotid arteries and the branches of the vertebral and basilar arteries. In an individual without significant blood vessel disease, approximately 70±10% of CBF is delivered by way of the internal carotid artery (anterior circulation), with approximately 30±10% supplied by the vertebral and basilar arteries (posterior circulation).

3. CBF is commonly described as the volume of blood in milliliters delivered to 100 gm of brain tissue per minute (ml/100 gm/min). Gray

matter receives more blood supply (65 to 180 ml/100 gm/min) than white matter (14 to 25 ml/100 gm/min). Calculated mean CBF = 55 ml/100 gm/min.

4. CBF is carefully regulated to ensure an adequate supply of glucose and oxygen to satisfy neuronal metabolic needs and consequently, normal neurologic function. Several mechanisms operate to maintain stable CBF despite fluctuations in systemic blood pressure and flow. The well-known regulatory mechanisms are commonly referred to as autoregulation, metabolic regulation, chemical regulation, and neurogenic regulation.

5. *Autoregulation* is a mechanism involving cerebral vascular smooth muscle that operates to maintain CBF at uniform levels in the face of changes in *mean arterial blood pressure* (MAP). When MAP rises, vessels (precapillary arterioles) constrict, restricting blood flow slightly, thereby maintaining CBF at fixed levels. When MAP decreases, vessels dilate, opening vessels slightly, thereby maintaining CBF at fixed levels. These mechanisms are effective in maintaining an adequate supply of blood to the brain when MAP is between 60 and 160 mm Hg, a range of pressures commonly referred to as the *regulatory plateau*. The pressures marking the regulatory plateau can be altered or "shifted" in response to sustained conditions such as chronic hypertension.

6. *Chemical regulation* refers to the mechanism whereby CBF is influenced by certain gasses, metabolic products, and pH. For example, conditions that result in an increase in arterial pCO_2 or a decrease in arterial O_2 will result in vasodilatation and an increase in CBF. An increase in serum lactate or pyruvate will also result in vasodilatation and an increase in CBF. A decrease in pH will result in vasodilatation and an increase in CBF.

7. *Metabolic regulation* refers to the mechanism whereby CBF is influenced by select, circulating ions. For example, conditions that result in an increase in circulating K+, H+, NO, and adenosine will result in cerebral vasodilatation.

8. *Neurogenic regulation* is the least effective of several mechanisms known to influence CBF and refers to intrinsic and extrinsic mechanisms involving nerve cells themselves. Intrinsic mechanisms involve the effect of certain cellular products on cerebral blood flow. For example, norepinephrine released by cells of the locus ceruleus can act to cause vasodilatation. Serotonin released by the raphe nuclei of the brainstem can act to cause vasoconstriction. Extrinsic mechanisms involve weak effects mediated by the autonomic nervous system. Sympathetic activation can result in weak cerebral vasoconstriction,

---

Table 7-1

Cerebral Blood Flow: Measurements, Calculations, and Determinations

	MEAN VALUES
MAP = diastolic BP + 1/3 (systolic BP – diastolic BP)	90±5 mm Hg
CPP = MAP – CVP	
$CBF = \dfrac{CPP}{CVR} = \dfrac{MAP - CVP}{CVR}$	85±5 mm Hg
	55 ml/100 gm/min

NORMAL RANGE VALUES

MAP – mean arterial pressure (ml/100 gm/min)	80 to 100 mm Hg
CPP – cerebral perfusion pressure (mm Hg)	75 to 95 mm Hg
CVP – cerebral venous pressure (mm Hg)	4 to 6 mm Hg
CVR – cerebrovascular resistance (mm Hg)	1.6 mm Hg
CBF – cerebral blood flow	55 ml/100 gm/min

---

whereas parasympathetic activation can result in weak vasodilatation.

9. Cerebral blood flow (ml/100 gm/min) is related to several measurable parameters of cerebrovascular function, including cerebral perfusion pressure (CPP), mean arterial pressure (MAP), cerebrovascular resistance (CVR), cerebral venous pressure (CVP), and cerebral blood volume (CBV). Changes in any of these values will affect cerebral blood flow and may result in the development of clinical signs and symptoms (Table 7-1).

10. Reduction in CBF can result in impairment or loss of neuronal and neurologic function. The cellular and clinical characteristics of the resulting abnormality are determined by several factors related to the speed of onset, duration, and magnitude of flow reduction; the size of the area involved; and the adequacy of collateral circulatory pathways.

11. The most common cause of brain dysfunction involving vascular mechanisms is ischemia. Functional (clinical) abnormalities develop when CBF is reduced to levels that provide the brain with inadequate

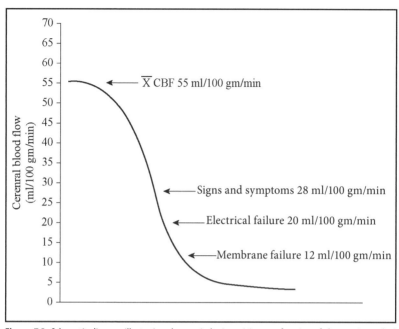

Figure 7-2: Schematic diagram illustrating changes in brain activity as a function of changes in cerebral blood flow.

amounts of oxygen and/or glucose. CBF reduction to approximately 28 ml/100 gm/min results in the development of signs and symptoms of neurologic dysfunction. Reduction to approximately 20 ml/100 gm/min results in *electrical failure* (ie, impaired ability to transmit nerve impulses). These are reversible effects that improve by increasing CBF to adequate levels. Reduction to approximately 12 ml/100 gm/min results in *membrane failure* (ie, impaired ability to deliver enough glucose and oxygen to maintain the function of the ion pumps within the cell membrane). Membrane failure is associated with the diffusion of intra- and extracellular ions down their concentration gradients. The resulting influx of sodium and chloride is accompanied by the obligatory intracellular accumulation of water. This is an irreversible effect that leads to infarction. An increase in intracellular water within neurons and glial cells is referred to as *cytotoxic edema* (Figure 7-2).

12. Because the brain has very limited energy reserves, sudden (acute) episodes of ischemia result very quickly in neuronal injury. Electrical failure occurs in approximately 10 seconds following global hypoperfusion. Membrane pump failure occurs at approximately 30 seconds.

Glucose and glycogen reserves are totally depleted by approximately 60 seconds with the development of irreversible cellular changes beginning at approximately 60 seconds following the total interruption of CBF.

13. Two mechanisms are commonly associated with failure to provide the brain with adequate amounts of oxygen and glucose: ischemia and hypoxia. *Ischemia* results from failure to deliver an adequate amount of blood to the brain. *Energy failure* is the result of inadequate brain perfusion. Ischemia is commonly described as focal or diffuse. Hypoxia results when inadequate amounts of oxygen are available to convert glucose into energy. Hypoxia can be caused by a reduction in blood oxygen content or oxygen-carrying capacity of the blood. Four different mechanisms of brain hypoxia are defined: *anoxic, anemic, histotoxic,* and *static.*

14. Neuronal cell death resulting from ischemia presents in several different ways depending on factors such as the size, duration, and mechanism of the ischemic injury. *Selective vulnerability* refers to a condition in which only certain types of cells are affected. In decreasing order of vulnerability, nerve cells are more vulnerable that astrocytes, which are more vulnerable that oligodendrocytes, which in turn are more vulnerable than brain endothelial cells. Among the most sensitive cells to ischemic insult are Purkinje cells of the cerebellum and pyramidal cells in Sommer's sector (CA 1) of the hippocampus. *Selective neuronal necrosis* refers to a condition in which only nerve cells are affected. *Laminar necrosis,* in which only certain cells of the cerebral cortex are affected, is an example of selective neuronal necrosis. *Pan-necrosis* refers to the condition in which ischemia affects all cells in the ischemic area. Pan-necrosis typically results in the formation of cavitary lesions in the brain.

15. Signs and symptoms associated with ischemia are determined chiefly by size and location of the ischemic area, the rate at which the ischemic episode progresses, the duration of ischemia, and the effectiveness of available collateral circulatory pathways and mechanisms. Clinically, the location of the ischemic area (infarct) can be determined by a careful evaluation of neurologic function (history, signs, and symptoms), focusing on both the neurologic functions that are impaired by the lesion as well as those that remain intact.

VENTRICLES AND CEREBROSPINAL FLUID

Key Points

1. The ventricles of the brain (lateral, third, and fourth ventricles) are the adult derivatives of the lumen of the embryonic neural tube. The ventricular cavity, like the functionally obliterated central canal of the spinal cord with which it is connected, is lined by a specialized epithelium composed of ciliated cuboidal cells known as *ependymal cells*. The ependymal cells, other than those associated with the CSF-producing choroid plexus, lack tight junctions. Thus, under certain conditions, CSF may cross the ependymal lining, typically into the periventricular regions of the brain.

2. The *choroid plexus* is a specialized secretory structure consisting of fenestrated capillaries derived primarily from branches of the anterior and posterior choroidal arteries together with the surrounding choroid epithelium (ependymal cells). Choroid plexus is found in the lateral, third, and fourth ventricles. Choroid epithelial cells are similar in morphology to the ependymal cells that line the ventricular cavity except that the choroid epithelial cells are joined by tight junctions. CSF is produced by the choroid plexus and released into the ventricular cavity. CSF production is not the result of passive diffusion or the filtration of plasma constituents but is rather the product of an active energy-requiring process involving the choroid epithelium. The process involves selective endocytosis by the choroid epithelial cells of substances that pass out of the choroidal capillaries through fenestra, synthesis within the choroid epithelial cell, and exocytosis from the apical side of the ependymal cell into the ventricular cavity. As long as the energy requirements of the choroid epithelial cells are satisfied, CSF will be produced. Increases in ventricular volume or pressure do not impair or reduce CSF production. CSF is produced at a rate of .35 to .37 ml/min or approximately 400 to 500 ml/day.

3. The ventricles contain approximately 20 to 25 ml of CSF in the "normal" individual.

4. CSF produced in the lateral ventricles flows through the foramen of Monro into the third ventricle, from which it passes into the fourth ventricle by way of the cerebral aqueduct (aqueduct of Sylvius). CSF then passes from the fourth ventricle into the subarachnoid space of the infratentorial compartment by way of the foraminae of Magendie

and Luschka. CSF produced in the fourth ventricle also passes through the two above-mentioned foraminae into the subarachnoid space of the infratentorial compartment.

5. Disease processes that restrict or obstruct the flow of CSF out of the ventricular compartment result in a buildup of CSF within the ventricular cavity and dilatation of the ventricles—a condition referred to as *obstructive* or *noncommunicating hydrocephalus*. The most common site of obstruction to flow within the ventricular system is at the level of the cerebral aqueduct. In such cases, the lateral and third ventricles will become dilated with no enlargement of the fourth ventricle. Intraventricular shunting procedures may be necessary to prevent significant neurologic injury and dysfunction resulting from a buildup of CSF within the ventricular system.

6. CSF within the skull is located in two distinct compartments: the ventricular compartment within the brain and the subarachnoid space surrounding the brain. The comparatively large subarachnoid spaces, particularly in relation to the brainstem, cerebellum, and hypothalamus are referred to as *cisterns*. Many of these cisterns can be visualized in neuroimaging studies and are therefore important in evaluating neurologic function. The volume of the intracranial cisterns (subarachnoid space) is approximately 80 to 85 ml. (Thus, the total volume of CSF within the cranial cavity is approximately 100 to 110 ml.)

7. CSF is free to move downward through the foramen magnum to occupy the spinal subarachnoid space. Approximately 25 to 30 ml collects caudal to the conus medullaris in the lumbar cistern, where it can be withdrawn (lumbar puncture) for diagnostic purposes.

8. CSF passing from the fourth ventricle into the subarachnoid space of the infratentorial compartment must eventually pass superiorly through the tentorial notch to enter the subarachnoid space of the supratentorial compartment. CSF in the supratentorial compartment occupies the subarachnoid space and ultimately passes through specialized structures of the arachnoid membrane known as arachnoid granulations. *Arachnoid granulations* are one-way valve-like structures that permit CSF to flow unidirectionally from the subarachnoid space into one of the dural venous sinuses. The capacity of the arachnoid granulations to transmit CSF from the subarachnoid space into the dural venous sinuses is approximately 4 to 6 times the rate of CSF production.

9. Some diseases such as meningitis can damage the arachnoid granulations and impair their function, resulting in a reduction in the

movement of CSF from the intracranial subarachnoid space into the dural venous sinuses. In such cases, CSF production may exceed CSF resorption, leading to an increase in intracranial volume and thus, *intracranial pressure* (ICP). In such cases, pressure on the brain will be increased both from the inside (because of increased CSF volume within the ventricles) and from the outside (because of increased CSF volume in the subarachnoid space). The resulting condition is referred to as *nonobstructive* or *communicating hydrocephalus.*

10. The optic nerve is a CNS structure, not a peripheral nerve as its name might suggest. As such, it is surrounded by meningeal layers, including the subarachnoid membrane and thus, the subarachnoid space. The subarachnoid space extends distally to the posterior margin of the eyeball. Increases in ICP are consequently transmitted through the CSF surrounding the optic nerve and can manifest as a bulging forward of the optic disc, resulting in papilledema.

INTRACRANIAL PRESSURE/ VOLUME RELATIONSHIPS

Key Points

1. The human brain resides within the rigid confines of the cranial cavity. The cranial cavity (cranial vault) is subdivided into compartments by thin sheets (*reflections*) of the dura mater. The major dural reflections, the falx cerebri and tentorium cerebelli, not only compartmentalize the cranial cavity, but also give structural support to other intracranial structures, including the dural venous sinuses. The anatomical relationship between the brain, the dura mater, and skull is both helpful (eg, protecting the brain from injury due to trauma) and harmful (eg, an abnormal increase in volume in one or more of the intracranial constituents).

2. The contents of the cranial cavity include 1) brain (neurons, glia, and intercellular fluid), 2) blood (distributed within the arteries, capillaries, veins, and dural sinuses), and 3) cerebrospinal fluid (distributed within the ventricles and subarachnoid cisterns) (Table 7-2). These three components exist in a dynamic, volume equilibrium in the normal condition. Sensitive mechanisms exist to maintain a stable intracranial volume and hence, a stable ICP. These mechanisms operate in accordance with the Monro-Kellie hypothesis (doctrine). The physiological purpose of these mechanisms is to maintain ICP at a stable level within the normal physiologic range in response to changes

Table 7-2		
Volume and Relative Contribution of the Three Major Intracranial Constituents		
BRAIN	**1400 ML**	**87%**
Cells (neurons, glia)	1190 ml	
Extracellular fluid (ECF)	210 ml	
BLOOD	**100 ML**	**6%**
Veins and dural sinuses	75 ml	
Arteries and capillaries	25 ml	
CEREBROSPINAL FLUID (CSF)	**105 ML**	**7%**
Ventricles	20 to 25 ml	
Intracranial cisterns	80 to 85 ml	
Total intracranial volume	1605 ml	100%

in intracranial volume. The Monro-Kellie hypothesis can be used to predict the consequences of increases or decreases in the volume of one or more of the intracranial components.

3. Normal brain function requires adequate supplies of oxygen and glucose, an efficient system for delivery of these substrates and removal of waste products, and efficient and effective mechanisms for regulating and responding to changes in intracranial volume and pressure. Several mechanisms exist for these purposes, mainly by altering and adjusting intracranial volume as a means of controlling ICP.

4. Normal ICP is 0 to 10 mm Hg, with 15 mm Hg being considered the upper limit of safety. Raised ICP is not harmful *per se* unless it leads to cerebral ischemia or contributes to pressure gradients and subsequent tissue displacement (*herniation*). Ischemia becomes a concern as ICP increases to levels approaching *cerebral perfusion pressure* (CPP).

5. Compliance, in relation to brain function, refers to the ratio of a change in intracranial volume to the resulting change in ICP. Compliance is said to be high when the compensatory mechanisms

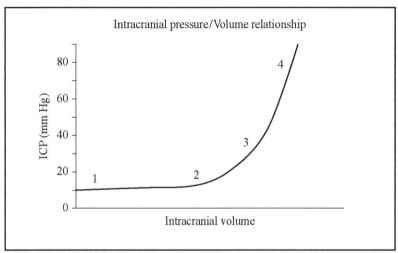

Figure 7-3: Schematic diagram illustrating the intracranial pressure/volume relationship.

function properly and low when the mechanisms function poorly or not at all. At normal intracranial volumes (approximately 1600 ml), ICP is typically within normal limits and will remain within the normal in the face of small, incremental increases in intracranial volume, a response suggesting that compliance is high and that compensatory mechanisms are functioning effectively. At normal intracranial volumes, these mechanisms are effective in preventing or limiting an appreciable increase in ICP. As intracranial volume increases further, additional compensatory mechanisms are activated in an effort to maintain ICP within normal limits. These mechanisms include the selective redistribution of intracranial content (Figure 7-3). As intracranial volume increases further, the compensatory mechanisms become less effective (or ineffective), with the result that incremental increases in intracranial volume will result in greater increases in ICP than at lower intracranial volumes. As intracranial volume increases even further, small incremental increases in intracranial volume will result in disproportionally large increases in ICP. In these later circumstances, when the compensatory mechanisms no longer function adequately, compliance is said to be low, and serious, sometimes life-threatening complications ensue.

6. Mechanisms for maintaining and stabilizing ICP generally involve mechanisms for altering intracranial volume. The first mechanism to be activated is displacement of CSF. CSF is initially displaced from the cisternal compartment through the foramen magnum. Other,

subsequently activated mechanisms are aimed at maintaining CBF at constant, stable levels in response to physiological and pathological changes in systemic blood pressure.

7. Conditions that result in blockage of the flow of CSF within the ventricular system or into the dural venous sinuses can result in an increase in intracranial volume and a consequent increase in ICP. Increases in intraventricular pressure can lead to movement of CSF across the ventricular ependymal lining into the periventricular regions of the brain, causing a condition referred to as *interstitial edema*. Shunting procedures may be necessary to manage these conditions.

8. Hemorrhage from a variety of causes and in a variety of locations will result in an increase in intracranial volume and ICP. Slowly accumulating volumes of extravascular blood, such as might be associated with bleeding from a torn bridging vein, may be compensated for effectively without significant changes in ICP. More rapidly accumulating volumes, such as might be associated with bleeding from an intracranial artery, may result in rapid increases in extravascular blood that overpower the compensatory mechanisms. These situations often result in pressure gradients within the cranial cavity that lead to brain herniation syndromes.

9. Reductions in CBF that lead to ischemic brain injury can also result in an increase in ICP. Ischemia involving neurons and glial cells may result in membrane ion pump failure, which in turn may lead to the movement of ions down their concentrations and the movement of water (intercellular fluid) into the cell. Brain swelling (edema) caused by the movement of water into cells from the extracellular compartment is referred to as *cytotoxic edema*.

10. Reduced CBF can also damage capillary endothelial cells and the BBB, leading to the movement of large serum protein molecules and water out of the vascular system, into the brain intercellular space. Edema caused by the movement of water from the vascular compartment into the intercellular compartment is referred to as *vasogenic edema*.

11. Sudden increases in intravascular pressure can overcome the cerebrovascular resistance, producing high pressure flooding of the capillary beds and a hydrostatic pressure gradient sufficient to drive water across the capillary wall into the extracellular space. The resulting increase in brain water is referred to as *hydrostatic edema*.

12. Marked reductions in serum osmolality, such as might be associated with hyponatremia, can result in diffuse brain swelling and raised ICP, a phenomenon referred to a *hypo-osmotic edema*.

13. Increases in intracranial volume sufficient to cause an increase in ICP will result in displacement of one or more of the intracranial contents as predicted by the Monro-Kellie hypothesis. Increases in ICP in the supratentorial compartment will commonly result in herniation of brain tissue from the region of higher pressure into a region of lower pressure. In the supratentorial compartment, herniation syndromes include subfalcine herniation, in which the cingulate gyrus on one side is forced medially beneath the inferior margin of the falx cerebri, with possible damage to the supracallosal segment of the anterior cerebral artery. More commonly, increases in ICP resulting from processes above the tentorium cerebelli will result in herniation of the uncus downward through the tentorial notch (*uncal herniation*). Uncal herniation frequently results in lateral displacement of the midbrain and compression of the ipsilateral oculomotor nerve. In some cases, the midbrain may by pushed firmly against the rigid edge of the tentorium cerebelli, resulting in an indentation of the midbrain in the region of the cerebral peduncle, a finding at autopsy commonly referred to a *Kernohan's notch*. Increases in ICP originating in the infratentorial compartment (posterior cranial fossa), commonly the result of hemorrhage into the cerebellum, can result in downward herniation of the cerebellar tonsil through the foramen magnum, a condition referred to as *tonsillar herniation*. Displacement of the cerebellar tonsil into the foramen magnum can result in compression of the caudal brainstem and uppermost cervical segments of the spinal cord.

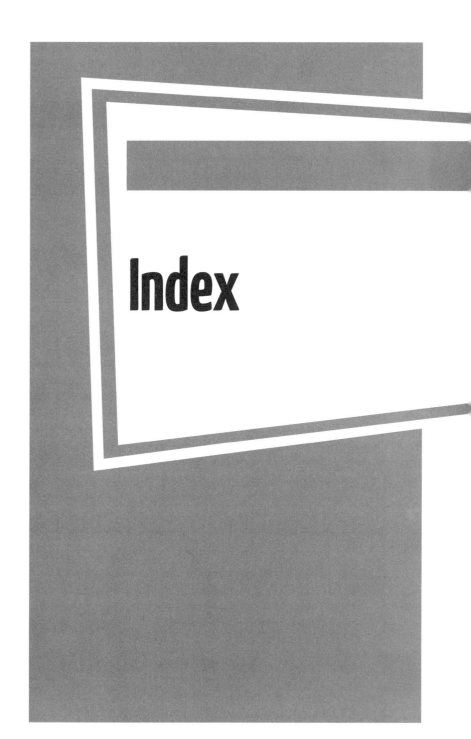

Index

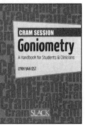
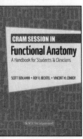

Attention Industry Partners!

Whether you are interested in buying multiple copies of a book, chapter reprints, or looking for something new and different — we are able to accommodate your needs.

MULTIPLE COPIES

At attractive discounts starting for purchases as low as 25 copies for a single title, SLACK Incorporated will be able to meet all of your needs.

CHAPTER REPRINTS

SLACK Incorporated is able to offer the chapters you want in a format that will lead to success. Bound with an attractive cover, use the chapters that are a fit specifically for your company. Available for quantities of 100 or more.

CUSTOMIZE

SLACK Incorporated is able to create a specialized custom version of any of our products specifically for your company.

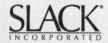